MW00800676

Magical Healing

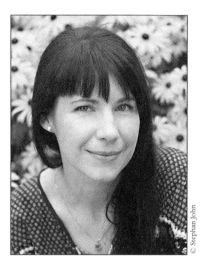

About the Author

Hi, my name is Claire. I am a witch, fortune teller, and author of several books on natural magic.

I was born in 1981 in the former German Democratic Republic, but now it is fortunately one Germany without any walls. As a child, I grew up in a rural environment with lots of folk customs and traditions (also magical ones) in a family with an almost hereditary passion for history, religions, and mythology.

Spirituality is nothing miraculous or detached to me. It simply means to communicate with the source of all things, that which moves and changes all forms of life, whether you call it God, Goddess, Spirit, or whatever you like. It's about all those things between heaven and earth who give that special magical spark to our lives.

Besides my work as an author, I also do readings (tarot, lenormand, and playing cards) and teach correspondence courses in German about natural magic and witchcraft.

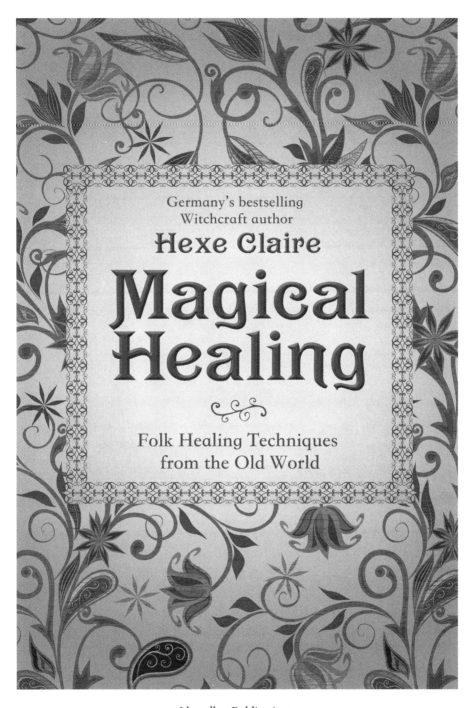

Germany's bestselling
Witchcraft author

Hexe Claire

Magical Healing

Folk Healing Techniques
from the Old World

Llewellyn Publications
Woodbury, Minnesota

First Edition
First Printing, 2018

Cover design by Shira Atakpu
Editing by Elysia Gallo and Brian Erdrich
Mano Figa Hand Charm on page 187 © Maxine Miller, used with permission
Translation by Hexe Claire and Maike Singelmann

Llewellyn Publications is a registered trademark of Llewellyn Worldwide Ltd.

Library of Congress Cataloging-in-Publication Data (Pending)
ISBN: 978-0-7387-5684-4

Llewellyn Worldwide Ltd. does not participate in, endorse, or have any authority or responsibility concerning private business transactions between our authors and the public.

All mail addressed to the author is forwarded but the publisher cannot, unless specifically instructed by the author, give out an address or phone number.

Any internet references contained in this work are current at publication time, but the publisher cannot guarantee that a specific location will continue to be maintained. Please refer to the publisher's website for links to authors' websites and other sources.

Llewellyn Publications
A Division of Llewellyn Worldwide Ltd.
2143 Wooddale Drive
Woodbury, MN 55125-2989
www.llewellyn.com

Printed in the United States of America

Other Books by Hexe Claire

Basiswissen Weiße Magie (Basics of White Magic)

Die Magie der Hexen (Witches Magic)

Kerzenmagie (Candle Magic)

Magie leben (Beyond Magic)

Das kleine Zauberbuch (The Little Book of Spells)

Magischer Hausputz (Magical Home Cleansing)

Stadthexen (Urban Witchcraft)

Magische Heilkunst (Magical Healing)

Contents

Preface:
The Old Arts of Healing

Gesundheit!

When it comes to magic, most people today think of love spells and money magic, but the magic of our forbearers was most often magic of healing.

The health and well-being of all inhabitants of a farm or house were the foundation for everything else. Times may change, but people's essential needs always stay the same.

Then as well as now our health is the most precious thing we possess, and often we become aware of it only when we lose what once seemed so natural.

I come from a family with an almost hereditary interest in all things of heaven and earth, so in my childhood it was normal to cure with herbs, magical words, and sometimes magical actions, but no one thought of them as "magical." It was just the way one did things in order to fix them quickly.

Later, in school and at college, I realized not everybody knew which tea to drink to get rid of certain ailments or that there are words that can do something beyond merely communicate.

I learned this when the others were astonished about my suggestions to use this tea or that herbal salve to cure something. Because this knowledge obviously appeared strange to some, I became more reticent about talking about those things (well, in your teen years you definitely don't want to look like an herb hag!).

When I came out of the spiritual closet with my work and began reading cards, writing esoteric books, and teaching courses, I still hid my interest in healing, as if my early experiences had stopped me from talking about that topic. But as time went on I recognized that times have changed.

Today many prejudices that were very common in my childhood are vanishing. Some hospitals are embracing traditional Chinese medicine, and no one is seen as an "esoteric weirdo" for getting acupuncture anymore.

I don't work as an herbal healer (and in Germany this is very strictly regulated when it comes to practitioners who are not medical doctors), but the needs of people made me search even more for the old knowledge, so I started remembering and compiling everything I could.

My approach is the happy medium: spirituality cares for the soul and the spirit, while common medicine cares for the body. Of course, in real life they merge. A spiritual or magical cure can increase our own self-healing powers, so that no pills are needed. Likewise, a much-needed surgery can balance not only the body, but also bring the soul and spirit of a patient back into harmony. Neither method is automatically better than the other; it always depends on the individual situation.

This book is also meant to express my deep respect for the last shamans of my own German culture, the wise women and men who still know how to "talk off" illnesses (which we'll explore later) and cure with the laying on of hands. They are often overlooked in the colorful circus of modern esotericism. They don't create new trends. They don't seek new methods all the time. They simply refer to the time-proven methods and tried and true knowledge that can sometimes be traced back for centuries and even millennia through historical findings.

But I want to do more than just to bring old traditions and healing knowledge to light. I also want to encourage you in your own abilities to heal. Often we tend to think that only others can help us: the doctor, the famous healer, or whoever. It is true that we humans need each other; the care and compassion of other people often helps to boost self-healing effects. But we also need to trust in ourselves and to take our personal responsibility seriously, especially when it comes to healing, because there is never just one way that suits everybody. When it comes to healing, knowledge is not only power, but the opportunity to make the best decisions for your own concerns.

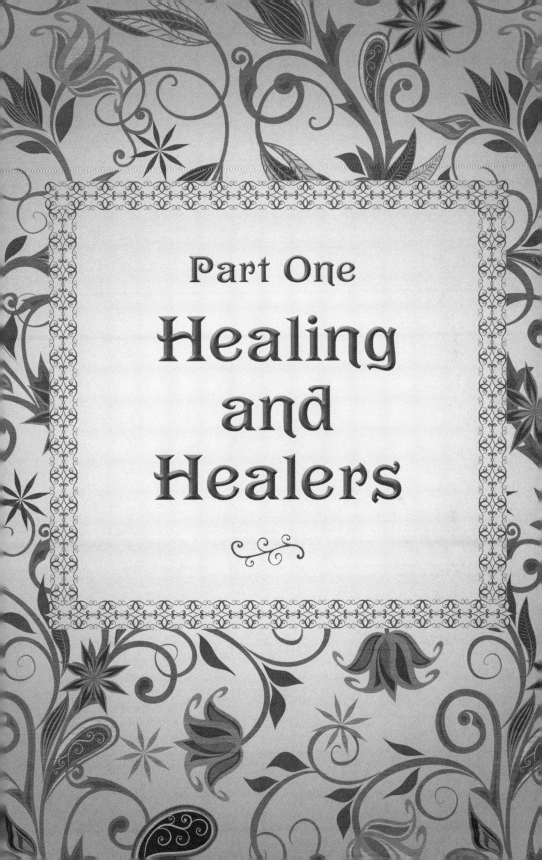

Part One
Healing and Healers

Healing, Past and Present

This book is about traditional cures as they were practiced by our ancestors. You may or may not have German or European ancestry, but anyone can explore and use the techniques in this book. Before we start, allow me to mention one or two things, if you would.

When it comes to forms of alternative or traditional healing, many people tend to look to Chinese, Indian, or Japanese traditions. Working with chakras, prana healing, reiki, and many other exotic modalities are very popular today. North or South American shamanic healing systems and African traditions are being further studied and investigated as well.

Viewed from the outside, the impression could arise that our region—Europe in general, or Germany in particular—had nothing of its own to contribute to the worldwide knowledge of healing. People seem to search for healing knowledge everywhere, but not right at their doorstep.

Of course, today we enjoy a worldwide exchange of ideas and knowledge, and there is nothing wrong with that. It's not that our own cultural knowledge is always better than things learned from others; such a view would be narrow-minded and arrogant. And what is "our own culture" anyway? Especially here in Europe with all the historical migrations and the exchange of ideas and traditions through trade routes, many traditional healing practices have similarities or are found in different variations but with the same core ideas across many regions.

If our ancestors had all the possibilities of the internet and modern media, they'd have certainly used it too. But it's also important not to overlook what we have here.

Our own traditions are often underestimated, and there are two reasons for this. First of all, people love exotic things. Things that are strange, extraordinary, and unfamiliar catch our attention more strongly than what we already know. Well, what we *think* we know. Whether we really know it thoroughly is another matter, but it's familiar to us at least.

The second reason is that many traditional practitioners are quite reserved when it comes to sharing their wisdom. As a result, it often dies with them, particularly if they find no suitable person to transmit it to who can carry on their work. Although healing is something that never goes out of demand, many traditional healers have difficulties finding the right person to train.

There is an enormous difference between the loud and sometimes dazzling world of healing workshops, seminars, and coaching on the one hand, and the more quiet and secretive world of traditional folk magic healers on the other.

The latter almost never appear in the media, and they mostly work in their surrounding areas. Often one only gets to know them by word of mouth and they are not very chatty about their art.

There are good reasons for this, of course, especially here in Germany due to strict legal restrictions in matters of healing. Even reasonable healers who always recommend seeing a doctor can face difficulties.

Some time ago the story of a farmer made the rounds through the media. He sold his products at a small traditional farmer's market and was also known by local people as someone who can cure with prayers. So, a woman plagued by headaches asked him to pray for her. The farmer did not make any promises to cure and he took no money from the woman, it was just a simple prayer. But a third person noticed this healing prayer and brought the farmer to trial for the illegal practice of medicine.

The farmer won the case, but this story makes clear why so many traditional healers only work in secret and demand absolute discretion from their clients.

Of course, the old images connected to healing are still alive. Some time ago I saw a commercial for a cold medicine in which a creature was shown, which our ancestors would have called an "on-squatter" (German: *Aufhocker*, a spiritual being that sits on your shoulders and causes you to feel heavily burdened and weak). The makers of the commercial put a computer-generated evil grey spirit on the shoulders of the actor to symbolically show the effect of a cold on you. Consciously or unconsciously, they were portraying an age-old image in matters of healing.

But many things have naturally changed as time has gone on. In the past, many healing spells and rituals were concerned with infectious diseases, healing wounds, and healing burns. Some of these troubles are not very common anymore, at least not in our part of the world. With major wounds and severe injuries, one goes to the doctor or the hospital. Modern medicines have taken away the terror of many infectious illnesses, and fresh foods in supermarkets give us vitamins and nutrients year-round, something our ancestors could only dream of.

The risk of injury has decreased significantly, or has changed in nature; for example, we didn't use to have car accidents. But who chops firewood or cuts grass with a scythe anymore? Not to mention doing laundry in big tubs heated over a fire and all the possible accidents that can happen with that. In the past a small carelessness could cause severe harm.

The healing magic of the olden days was often about those crisis situations: to stanch blood, to cool burns immediately, to relieve pain, and to help wounds to heal without scarring. In those days one could not call 911, a doctor was seldom available in the vicinity, and even if one was, his treatments often were unaffordable for ordinary people.

And of course, the standard of knowledge has increased. Our ancestors were not as simple as many people think, but many things were simply not known to them. For example, it makes a huge difference if you know about viruses and bacteria or not. But it's a strange coincidence that old drawings of demons of illnesses look quite similar to what is found under a microscope.[1] Today we still have sayings about beings causing an illness like having a frog in the throat or the German word for gout, *Zipperlein*; "Zipper" was an old word for dwarf.

Modern medicine has relieved us of many burdens. But are we truly happier or healthier? Not necessarily. This is because every era has its own challenges.

In the old days infections and the lack of surgical help were major problems. Today we have stress-related illnesses, allergies, skin problems, and cardiovascular diseases. And of course, we often tend to think how good things were in the good old days. This is often more a question of faith.

Take for example the famous glacier mummy called Ötzi, who lived about 5,200 years ago. It turns out even he had cardiovascular diseases and arteriosclerosis, something we think of today as a modern disease related to relative affluence. We can be sure Ötzi ate no fast food, but lived a healthy life. You see: we don't become perfect or indestructible just by following a "healthy lifestyle" (whatever that means at the given moment).

Because what is "healthy"? If you look back in history, so many things have been considered to be healthy without a doubt; one day, when we're history, people may smile about our ideas of healthy living.

In old cookbooks sugar is often praised as the best and purest form of energy, and therefore very healthy. Some experts recommended eating only steamed meals while others insisted on raw foods. Many spices—today favored because of their phytonutrients—were frowned upon because they would overexcite the body and harm it. Times are changing and, with them, our views on many topics.

Today some health trends are reminiscent of the sale of indulgences in the past, as new and exotic miracle plants, superfoods, diets, or exercises promise a healthy (eternal?) life. Healthy living is for many people a new kind of religion, with its angels (raw food, vegan, green smoothies, and similar buzzwords being fashionable right now, but always sub-

---

1. See the works of Wlislocki in the bibliography.

ject to rapid change), its demons (like sugar and fat), and with aspiration of salvation (if you are good) from the evils of, for example, aging or being the "wrong size." But of course, other things are also important when we look at the wide fields of health today. In German we call treatments *Behandlung*. The word *hand* appears inside the word, which refers to the body part just like in English, implying that patients will be touched by a doctor, who, aside from examining what's going on, also gets a hands-on feeling for the constitution of a person. Today most *Behandlungen* don't deserve the name. There's a lot of hecticness in most doctor's practices and sometimes there's not even time for a handshake between patient and doctor. Many doctors spend more time with administrative tasks than with their patients.

Over-motivated or badly performed fitness exercises do harm to joints, tendons, ligaments, and muscles, but often in such a subtle way that one doesn't realize and instead pays the price for it ten or twenty years later. Physiotherapy practices are full of people who overdid their sports. All those hurting jogging knees, yoga hips, or tennis arms didn't come from nothing, they were gained through hard work.

Taking certain vitamins and dietary supplements can sometimes harm more than help, and the border between "I just care about what foods I put into my body" and an eating disorder can be quite thin.

One does not need to be an expert to see that we live in a time of superlatives for everyone. It seems everyone is expected to be perfect and flawless. It's important to deal with that consciously, for no one lives in a vacuum. Every day we all see retouched pictures of perfect-looking humans—a nonverbal demand to reach the same status, but of course without the favors that Photoshop grants.

Illnesses today are often experienced as personal failure: something one is guilty of or could have prevented if one was "better," "trying harder," and so on.

There's a lot of pressure on today's sick person, and modern mystics often don't serve as shining examples in that matter, either, for example: if they babble about karmic debts or other kinds of failings immediately. As if the illness weren't bad enough on its own!

A little humor is also never out of place when it comes to this topic. A while ago I overdid it with jogging (you see, I also had to learn the hard way). After this my knee went on strike. I could only walk very slowly when out on the street—that is if I made it down the stairs first! Seniors would zoom past me with their wheeled walkers, and this is no joke. I was as slow as a snail.

One time a woman that I didn't even know personally told me I had huge karmic debts that were causing my knee problems. I told her with a wink, as I am wont to do, "It's not karma, it's cartilage!" Of course, she did not find that funny.

Never underestimate power plays when it comes to healing. If one is ill, weak, and maybe a bit confused, some people see this as an opportunity to push their egos and feel bigger than they really are.

The old magical healing systems of our region don't deal with karmic debts or things like that. It's more comparable to shamanic healing methods. The basic assumptions of traditional German/European healing are: here is an illness, it harms this person, so it has to be taken out and chased off so that it doesn't come back. There is no implication of "it's all your fault," "you're wrong," or impure, stupid, insolent, lazy, (insert your adjective here), and a terrible hedonist on top of it all.

Of course, traditional healers also speak frankly with their patients when they eat too much, don't exercise, or do similar things that diminish their life force. But they do this based on common sense and not to guilt-trip them or create dependencies. The basic principle is always that the illness is the evil, not the patient.

Karma and its associated concepts come from the Indian and Asian culture where they are deeply rooted in the life and spirituality of the local people. Our indigenous healing tradition has different roots and concepts.

The traditional spiritual helpers of our culture are God, Mary, Jesus, and the saints (and of course all the older gods and goddesses gleaming through them), as well as pre-Christian nature, plant spirits, and the energies of certain places, stones, trees, springs, rivers, and much more.

Later in the book we will see in detail how to adapt the old healing spells for modern times and your individual spiritual path, but this must be pointed out right from the start: it makes a huge difference whether an ill person feels like a guilt-burdened karmic sinner or like a regular human in need, who in spite of all their human deficiencies—or maybe precisely because of them—can rely on help from above.

Another point we must keep in mind when it comes to historical healing techniques is the trap of idealization. For example, one sometimes hears glorified stories about the "power-herbs of women in ancient times," where they used toxic plants for abortions like ergot. How many women died or sustained permanent damage from using these plants is never mentioned and maybe not even thought about.

Modern alternative healers sometimes also tend to divide our healing ancestors into "good" healers and midwives and their enemies, the "bad" doctors and pharmacists. But it's a fact that doctors also helped to preserve magical healing knowledge, as exemplified by the famous German occultist Siegfried Seligman in his 1922 classic about the magical power of the eyes (German title: *Die Zauberkraft des Auges*). Some doctors worked with magical and medical cures at the same time and many a pharmacist published sheets and small booklets with magical healing spells and herbal knowledge not all that long ago. The rift between traditional healers and doctors was not as deep as many assume it today. At least not always, and not everywhere.

Good healers have also always known that there are no across-the-board cures for everyone, because every person is different from others and even from themselves due to personal changes. Today advice is often given like, "You *have* to try this. It works!" Some people even get a little huffy when someone doesn't take their advice. But it is not that simple. Only with knowledge, intuition, and sometimes even trial and error can one find what is needed (and this is also true for academic medicine). By now it is well known that conventional drugs also work differently for every person. Some people face many adverse side effects while others face almost nothing. Every person is different.

Would you drink coffee to prevent insomnia? Certainly not. But this was exactly what the family doctor recommended to a friend of mine. Her blood pressure was quite low and that could hinder her body from falling asleep. The coffee cure worked and proved that even the simplest assumptions—like coffee being a "pick-me-up"— are not true for everyone.

Another friend of mine had a mouth guard to stop her from grinding her teeth at night, but her problem became even worse and her entire jaw was painfully tensed up. A physical therapist later told her that sometimes the body wants to re-establish the original alignment of the teeth in sleep and will unconsciously bite even harder when asleep to get rid of the foreign object.

We see that what's good for someone can cause problems for another person. These are two randomly selected situations, but they illustrate clearly how important it is to see every person as a unique individual and respect the natural differences between human bodies.

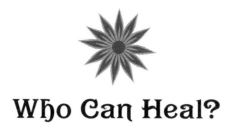

Who Can Heal?

Does everyone possess the inner ability to heal? Or does one need to be chosen, endowed with special powers, or have a certain personality? Sooner or later everyone interested in spiritual healing will stumble across this question.

What would the healers of the olden days have said to this? As to be expected, opinions differed a lot. But one essential credo was always the same: everyone who has a firm belief in healing and truly wants to can heal. This has a little catch: the proper form of wanting must be mastered first. So, what did our forbearers mean by "wanting"?

They were not referring to a blindfolded will that says, "This simply has to work out!" Most healers were (and are) very spiritual persons who knew that the final say is up to the spiritual forces of life. No traditional healer would have claimed to have this healing power. The traditional healer does not heal on their own. A healer in the old sense is a medium for the forces of life that can restore balance to the ill person. This is a very important point. Real healers have no hubris.

Of course, healers also have different temperaments. Some have an open and chatty manner, some are very calm, while others can be rather abrupt and direct in their behavior. And more than a few of them tend to enjoy little pranks. As different as they may be, they all know that the powers that be are the true source of power when healing comes about.

This means one not only needs the powerful desire to heal but also a deep trust in the powers of good, or more precisely, the powers of balance.

Traditional healing systems all over the world see illnesses as a kind of falling out of balance. Illness is a disequilibrium that can be cured when balance is restored. Healers need an imperturbable belief that healing is possible (and this means *possible*, for no human is almighty).

The people seeking advice or treatment are often not so sure whether it will really help, but this is not a necessary requirement in traditional healing. An old prayer healer put it this way: "When they come to me they already believe, otherwise they would not be here."

For modern people, it can seem quite archaic to distinguish so clearly between good versus evil as our ancestors did. I use these terms because they are common in our native healing tradition. People in those days did not vacillate as much as we do. A spade was called a spade, as all shamanic cultures still call it. Today we might instead speak of harmony versus blockages. The healers of the old days also knew that the illness is not evil, per se, but it is evil when it's in the body of someone, harming this person; therefore, it must be taken out—making no bones about it.

When you start to embrace the old knowledge please feel free to experiment with it and adapt it. We live today, and not everything that was suitable in the past is appropriate now. Nevertheless, I have to insist that the old clear and direct way of speaking about illnesses has a power of its own.

If one says frankly "this is bad—it has to go away," one develops a whole different attitude than would be the case if first discussing it at length and losing oneself in looping thoughts. The power has to be bundled, kept together, and used purposefully; that's how magic worked and still works.

Of course, that's not to say one shouldn't think about an illness, consider their own role in it and the possibility they have to change things (like lifestyle habits, for example). But the outstanding effectiveness of the old healing spells has its roots in a clear definition of negative and positive, and knowing without a doubt what was to be achieved. When it is time to get down to business and looping thoughts are left behind, the focus concentrates solely on the restoration of balance.

But let's get back to the question of who is able to heal. Today we often think of healers as people who were somehow different or special, maybe a lovable eccentric, a grumpy old lady, or even a dynamic healer with powerful charisma.

Although there were some lovable eccentrics for sure, most healers were ordinary people next door. They had their day job or farm, and everybody in the village knew, for example, that neighbor Mr. Müller can cure this, and Mrs. Meier at the other end of the village knows how to get rid of that. If an illness caught you, you went to Mr. Müller or Mrs. Meier and were helped. Healing took place in the neighborhood, where people knew each other personally and everyone knew that he or she has this special gift, but apart from that is a normal person just like everyone else.

Today this has changed a lot. Of course, there still are the hidden working healers in small communities that outsiders won't ever hear of. But instead of them, most people interested in traditional healing will see more showy and self-promoting people at esoteric fairs and healing conferences. One needs a lot of luck to find a true healer at places like this. I know a couple of people who spend respectable sums on the stars of this media-friendly arranged healing scene without any bettering of their situation. This was also an impetus for this book because it would be wonderful if people would learn again to treat each other with mutual love and respect, without show-off healers, simply from human being to human being.

If you want to find out which healing abilities were given to you, there has to first be the opportunity to try it out. There has to be room to meet others without the pressure to succeed. There will be some trial and error but that's the way it is: experiences can only be made; they cannot be learned.

Of course, financial interests should not be the driving force for this. With traditional healers it's customary even nowadays to give them money in a small bowl in their home—unsolicited and as much as one wants to pay. Since everyone knows each other in small communities, no one will take advantage of the healer, and some thankful people leave even bigger sums.

This is a whole different situation compared to someone who tries out his or her healing abilities only to make money. In the old days most healers had their regular income not in the healing field but on their farm or their job. They did not depend on the healing financially.

This is an important point because it can be a drawback. If one wants to make a living from healing, one gets into a dependent situation. No errors are allowed anymore (and even the best doctors make errors) because it could damage their reputation and compromise their income. This leads to pressure, and pressure hinders the ease that is essential to spiritual healing.

Doing things with ease is the key to awakening the healing powers within. Some time ago a friend of mine and her partner treated each other. He had a persistent cough, and she had a rash. For the fun of it, both performed "magical" actions they invented spontaneously. He blew on her rash and symbolically swept it away with his hands. She made a gesture as if extracting his cough and threw it out of the window. Although (or because?) they did not take this seriously, it worked wonderfully for both of them.

We can learn something important from this couple. Everyone is able to heal when the energy is allowed to flow freely. Some can heal more easily than others (as we are all differently equipped with talents in different areas), but everyone has at least a spark of it.

Because my friend and her partner acted just for fun, both were free of expectations and blockages. They did not ask themselves, "Is it possible? Am I capable of doing this? Will I make a fool of myself? Will I look silly if it shows no effect?"

If one takes a playful approach toward spiritual healing, then there is nothing to lose and much to win.

This was not different in the old days. Many healers discovered their healing abilities by accident. Of course, there also were traditional healer families that passed on their knowledge (and not incidentally, the confidence to heal) from one generation to another. And often healers searched at the end of their lives for a student to pass on their knowledge to. But in the end it was not important how one started rather how well it worked.

In the healing context there is also the question: Do I need a healer? Can't I heal myself? Is this not true personal responsibility?

Yes and no. It's definitely a good choice to take responsibility for oneself, care for oneself, and get information while not putting it all on a healer. Many people unfortunately develop a passive dependency toward doctors or miracle healers.

On the other hand, one sometimes needs an impulse from the outside to get the ball rolling. There is a West African saying that says you can't give yourself the advice that helps you. With support from others there is more helpful energy and impetus for healing, which can make it a lot easier. One has a companion for the journey and doesn't have to figure out everything on one's own. This helps to save energy for the actual healing.

Most people visiting traditional healers don't expect miracles (at least in rural areas; in towns this can be different). This attitude also helps the healer, because healers have to be convinced of their abilities, yet at the same time they also know that they are not all-powerful. One has to meet each other simply as human beings without unrealistic expectations on the part of the patient but also without healers that glorify themselves.

Second Sight and Healing

In the past, healers were often credited with having second sight and being able to perceive spirits. This seems to mirror ancient shamanic ideas; if an illness is thought of as a harmful spiritual intruder, then a healer needs to be able to spot them to expel the illness. In other words, she or he has to have second sight.

There are these negative, consumptive spirits, but there are also helpful forces that are perceived by the traditional healer and with whom she or he works together, just as indigenous shamans do with their helping spirits (in fact, the expression "helping spirit" doesn't do justice to the power of these beings).

Many legends remind us to this day of this sacred bond between humans and spirits. This old knowledge might be encoded in myth and fairytales, but it still gleams and can be found. For example, there are many legends about healers who received their gift to heal from a fairy or an otherworldly encounter. Our ancestors believed that in spiritual healing many things happen in the energetic plane, the world of instinct and helpful forces.

The traditional Romany healer Hartiss put it this way: "You have to know that true healers can't learn any methods. A healer is like a painter, a sculptor or a musician. You know him by the work he performs."[2]

But the gift alone is not enough. One has to learn, and one has to work wholeheartedly. Even if someone has a natural sensitivity for healing, this person is still just a diamond in the rough.

Second sight, intuition, or however one wants to call it can't be learned, it is a gift. But the individual portion that was given to every one of us can be whetted and polished. To take the metaphor further, a big but unpolished diamond won't ever sparkle and shine as brightly as a small one that's been perfectly cut.

A spiritual gift is no blank check. All traditional cultures consider those gifts as a disposition. With practice and training, this disposition can blossom, but it can also slumber if we choose not to use it.

Basically, every person has at least a little spark of healing power. Persons with a bigger amount of it are able to heal to a larger extent. Or, put simply, not everyone will be good at math, but everyone can put two and two together.

---

2. Derlon, *Heiler und Hexer (Healers and Warlocks)*, 24

Matters of Attitude

In the old days healers often worked in their immediate vicinity where everyone knew each other. Today, however, this is very different. Many people approach healers with a consumerist mentality. "I give you this money, and you make me healthy again." This attitude causes many problems for healers.

I've often heard from healing practitioners that they are expected to do miracle healings in next to no time and with no contribution on the part of the patient—and at absolute bargain prices, please. Maybe this is a typical German attitude; other cultures do show much more respect for the skills of traditional healers.

Some people know the price of everything but the worth of nothing. The doctor Martina Bühring, who did a survey about Berlin's traditional healers, mentioned two examples that illustrate this issue clearly. In the first example, a woman went to a traditional healer to talk off her shingles and paid for two scheduled sessions in advance. After the first session she was cured of this wearisome and painful illness, but what did she do? She demanded the money for the second session back.

On another occasion, an Eastern European woman went to this healer to treat her migraine. Five sessions were scheduled, but she was also cured after the first one. And what did she do? In appreciation and thankfulness, she sent the healer the money for the other four sessions that were originally planned.

Another healer in Bühring's survey put it in a nutshell:

"Healing has much to do with the faith of a patient. Because of that, it works much faster when I treat foreigners (Poles, people from the former Yugoslavia) than Germans. Sometimes their illnesses vanish immediately.

"When it comes to Germans and especially Protestants, the healing process takes much more time. Polish people and people from other cultures believe in 'miracle healings' and they collaborate in the healing process. Their whole kin supports them, all of them pray together. Germans don't fight [for their health]. They go to the doctor first and often don't want to recover strongly enough. Their motto is: Now do something for your money."[3]

If there are no associations or gatherings for them, many healers in major cities plow a lonely furrow. In the olden days, when healing was a village business, respect was a matter of course, although in some regions healers were also seen as a bit eldritch (because, as they say, the one who can work for good can also work for evil). People knew each other and, most importantly, they had faith. This does not refer to faith in any specific religion, but a faith that there exists healing and helpful forces that we can work with to get relief or healing. In other words, a faith in the helpful forces of nature and the body that can be approached to activate self-healing powers.

Today this is often very different. Many patients are curious or don't go to a healer until everything else has failed and their situation has greatly worsened. In this state, they expect miracles from healers.

If you talk to healers, you will often hear the words "If only people would come sooner!" But many decide to go to healers only if it's bad enough to try "something like this." The despair that moves them doesn't have much in common with the faith of patients in the old days. Because of that, some healers ask their patients first if they have faith; if that's not the case, they send them away. One can't blame them for that. Who wants to waste time and energy on people who don't collaborate or "don't want to recover strongly enough" as the healer cited above put it?

---

3. Bühring, 67

Another problem that must be kept in mind (especially the western mind) when it comes to the activation of self-healing powers is over-analyzation. This often happens when people want to have guarantees and logical explanations for anything that happens, because they do not have faith in things that go beyond analytical thinking.

But no one can guarantee healing, no healer and no doctor. Instead of taking what Mother Nature gives us in the form of herbs or trusting the experience of a healer and her hands, they want reasons and justifications. The analytical mind picks it apart and pigeonholes until all the magic is gone.

Many legends also refer to this propensity, so it seems to be nothing new. The hero of a story is warned to not turn around after a magical happening; he turns around nevertheless and ruins everything. Or, for example, a woman knows she should not spy on the good house spirits but does so in spite of herself, and the little people leave her house forever. There are many more examples like this, all illustrating the point that over-analyzing or too closely examining the magical and enchanting sphere will cause it to lose its power.

Healing starts not in the domain of rational thinking. Healing starts in the deeper levels, the nonverbal levels, the realm of feelings, inner images, and our bodily sensations. From shamans to travelling Romany healers and from Low German hexers to southern Germany "turning" healers (we will come to that special healing technique in detail later in the book), they all know that the initial spark for healing comes from the depth of nonverbal perceptions.

In this context it is often said that we as humans have to tap into our animal nature to get in touch with the elemental force in every one of us.

Children are often much easier to treat because they embrace the healing energies naturally and don't over-analyze everything. Of course, children also ask: "What is this? What is it good for?" But when you explain it to them, they join in with enthusiasm.

A mother told me some time ago about her daughter, who had a cold. In addition to the prescribed medicines, she gave her daughter a pink dyed stone and told her it was a fairy stone that helps people get well. The little girl of course loved the color (and for a child it's irrelevant if a healing stone was dyed or naturally that way). It was pink and beautiful and appealed to her from the first moment. The little lady was so happy that her self-healing powers quickly increased, and she recovered faster than with other colds before.

The illness was "turned." The old turning healers couldn't have done it better. (As stated before, we will cover this technique at greater length later. In German what I'm calling "turning" is expressed with the word *wenden,* and people who practice this are called *Wender* or *Wenderin* because they have the ability to bring an illness to the turning point—the point from which then on it gets better.)

So, what should hinder us from becoming a child again for a moment when it can help us so much? Children indulge in their feelings and see the world with open senses, without the rational mind short-circuiting the process or putting the brakes on.

Please don't get me wrong. Rational thinking has an important role, too. You need it to make good decisions, collect the information you need, and evaluate it. But from the moment you've decided on your chosen path, physical perception should take the lead and our brooding mind should step back a bit. This, more than anything else, helps our self-healing powers to unfold and work for us, strong and unimpeded.

This is also the reason why many healers insist that their patients not thank them. The phrase "thank *you*" disturbs the *self*-healing powers. Traditional healers always have a fine sense for those tiny but important details. If someone says "thank you" to a healer, this indicates that the healer did all the work. But healers are impulse-givers. The rest is done by the faith and of course the immanent powers of the body of the patient. To root this deeply in the consciousness of their patients, the words "thank you" are taboo to many traditional healers.

Perils and Risks

Healing is a challenge. And this is not only true for the patient but also for the healer. If healers lack the ability to set boundaries or don't take enough time for their own regeneration, this is a risk.

In the old days this was known as the "jumping over" of an illness. This meant that if a healer didn't protect himself or set boundaries (for example, with symbolic cleanings the healer keeps a certain inner distance from the patient) he ran the risk of developing the same disease as the patient.

This is not just a fairytale or fable, as I've found while working on this book. A friend of mine had a persistent rash on her hands and would not let up, asking me, "Can't we try one of these spells you are collecting for your new book?" I refused at first, for after all, I'm a witch, not a professional healer. But she insisted that it couldn't hurt to try, so why not? She doesn't live near me (we will talk more about distance healing later in the book, as it was also practiced by our ancestors for several reasons), so I spoke the spells over a cell phone photo of her hands (you have to go with the times, right?). Because we are close friends, I never thought about setting boundaries.

The cure worked wonderfully, but a week later I had a red dot on my wrist and some days later it had grown to the size of a five-cent coin that looked exactly like the rash of my friend. I was laughing because it was too funny; a witch like me forgot to protect herself. I then told the rash to rush away, and everything turned out fine.

This is also an important point. Say what you want, but don't exaggerate anything. Trust yourself and your body to do its job.

Overwork is also a reason for illnesses to "jump over." Some of the famous Mexican folk healers (who are sometimes venerated like saints, so we know many stories of their lives) didn't even reach the age of thirty because they exhausted themselves in their work.

Every healer is different and so everyone must know his or her own limits—and respect them. I heard of a north German healer who has to rest after each patient for at least two hours. If someone comes along during this time for a healing session, they have to wait until the two hours are up.

Most healers treat at maximum five or six patients a day. Of course, there are exceptions; some people can treat twenty or more persons per day and feel great. Others treat only one or two patients, and there is nothing wrong with that. This is completely individual and the only thing that is important is to be true to oneself about it.

Someone who can see twenty patients per day is not "stronger" or "better" than someone else. This person is just built differently in the way their inner path of energy flows.

Of course, the topic of protection is not only relevant to traditional healers. Doctors and therapists are also well advised to take care of themselves and to find their own rituals or habits to create a healthy distance, so the illnesses of their patients don't jump over to them or undercut their strength. It's old knowledge that being in contact with illnesses every day can't be healthy—unless one protects oneself well.

To cite doctor Martina Bühring and her study again:

Classical doctors' traditional protection is a starched white coat.[4] But if this protection was sufficient, why do so many family doctors die from heart attacks quite early and why do so many psychiatrists commit suicide? There are many examples of somatic

---

4. In German the word "starched" is the same word as "strengthened." This is deliberate wordplay.

transfer. For example, many people start scratching when someone next to them reveals an itching skin disease. An example of psychological transfer is depressive patients who lower the vigor of the people around them.

What does this mean for the healer? He has to be able to empathize with the symptoms of the patient, to let the signals "come in." But he also has to be able to process these signals in a way that evokes no disease manifestation in him. This must be a dynamic process which enables the healer to keep his own body healthy.

Interestingly, certain healers can handle and "process" certain illnesses, while sending other illnesses on to other colleagues. This phenomenon can also be observed in hospitals, where certain doctors, consciously or unconsciously, provide help for a certain clientele by acting as contact persons.[5]

In the old days most healers worked more as specialists and not so much as general practitioners. Some took off pain, others worked as herbalists, some healed burns, and others stanched blood. One was able to talk off warts, others "the Rose" (skin infections and rashes). No one was surprised that healers were specialists who did not treat other illnesses because they knew their limits well.

Today healers are often expected to be able to treat any illness and many healers expect this from themselves too.

The way of our ancestors can be very inspiring in that matter. Being a specialist not only can prevent exhaustion, but it also helps to get a real deep knowledge of your area of expertise.

Creating routines helps to develop a healer's individual system, step by step. (We will cover this later in more detail, because healing should be embedded in a system in some ways.) Healers who know well their spiritual guides, their helpers (stones, plants, gestures, spells, etc.), and

---

5. Bühring, S., 53

their abilities—but also their limits—won't be knocked off their feet easily.

But if someone is uncertain, has no overall context for the healing work, or tries out new systems all the time, they won't be able to raise sufficient healing power for the longer term, gradually leeching themselves out over time. If they also neglects their protection or simply work too much, this might even lead to damage.

In traditional societies shamans often learn to heal themselves first during their so-called initiatory illness (also called shamanic crisis or shamanic illness; it's often a near-death experience or life-threatening illness that grants them special knowledge). This always comes first before they learn to heal anyone else.

Of course, there is no perfect human being anywhere—someone who has no problems and is always perfectly balanced. That's not what this is about. But one must at least be stable and powerful enough to be able to absorb the energies of the ill person during the healing procedure.

Being first able to heal oneself is like a safety net for the healer, so they can trust in their own ability to quickly get rid of an illness that jumps over.

Methods of Protection

The most important tool to prevent the jumping over or transference of illnesses is a healthy inner distance during the healing. Some people need no aids at all for this because they already have a healthy inner border that can be only shattered when they overwork.

But not everyone is this lucky and not without reason. A lot of the ability to heal comes from the ability to let in and literally empathize with the other who feels ill (empathy comes from the Greek word *empátheia*, which means "feeling into somebody," so naturally it blurs the boundaries between healer and patient).

Imagine the energy of the healer as a white cloud. During the healing procedure it wanders to the patient, intermixes with his or her energy and goes back to the healer, who reads out the information gained during the encounter. In practice this can happen quite quickly. Some healers see in split seconds what's wrong with the patient.

Healers with a mediumistic nature often even know who will show up next at their door with which problem. There are many true stories about healers that greeted their surprised incoming patients at the door with the appropriate herbal remedy for their illness.

To return to the cloud analogy above, their energy system is so sensitive that they feel what is in the air and know what weather front is approaching (this often merges with the ability of second sight).

Due to this sensitiveness healers can face two problems. The first one is that if he doesn't retrieve his cloud completely from the patient, he loses energy that leeches out. The patient gets a short energy boost from this but later returns to their previous energy level because this was just energy gained from the healer, not an impulse to generate new energy oneself.

This aspect is especially important for inexperienced healers, because this first improvement of the patient through catching the energy of the healer can start an unhealthy cycle between them. The healer gives his own energy and the patient takes it and feels a short-term improvement of his situation. But a real change does not happen, because a real change would mean an impulse to activate the self-healing forces in a patient to open his own sources of energy again. Healers that exhaust their energy in this way won't have enough for themselves one day.

Because of this, one of the most important principles of spiritual healing is to never work with your own energy, always let the healing forces of nature work through you. In fact, healing is the task of an intermediary. The healer gets in touch with a source of healing (through prayer, herbal knowledge, letting the energy flow through his hands, working with power animals or whatever is practiced in their culture) and lets the energy of this source flow to the patient. He's like a connecting cable, but he never is the source of this energy.

The second issue is letting go of the information and energies that were received by the patient after the treatment. If a healer neglects the inner cleansing—not cleaning up the exploratory cloud used to feel what's going on in the patient—he will eventually carry all the sorrows and hardships of his patients in an unfiltered way and his pure white cloud will become dirty and disheveled.

Of course, this applies not only to traditional healers, but also to doctors, therapists, nurses, healing practitioners, and spiritual consultants in general. All of them will benefit from observing those two things: taking their own energy back to themselves consciously, and cleansing it before incorporating (this is meant literally; *in corpus* means "into the body") it again.

Restoring the Energy

In many cases visualization is the best tool to bring the energy back to its original state after it was used to detect what's wrong with the patient. When the treatment is over, visualize taking back your energy cloud through your solar plexus and sealing it there.

The solar plexus plays an important role in many healing traditions worldwide. Of course, it's called many different names, but it's always that same spot in the body, about a hand's breadth under the heart. It is one of the most important plexuses in the human body; a hard strike to this region can lead to reflexogenic cardiac arrest.

If one prefers to work with more metaphorical visualizations, one can also imagine a little washing machine at the height of the solar plexus, pulling in and cleansing the small cloud thoroughly until it's clean and fresh again. One does not have to use stilted pictures or symbols for that; what works, works!

After difficult cases or when you are not fit as a fiddle it can be very helpful to frame the restoring of energy more tangibly—for example, with the help of a stone. The many varieties of quartz crystals are favored healing stones all over the world: agate, rock crystal, onyx, jasper, aventurine, rose quartz, carnelian, tiger's eye, citrine, amethyst, smoky quartz, or chalcedony. They can be wonderful helpers and are easy to use. Lay a quartz crystal on your solar plexus, and imagine your little cloud coming back to you filtered through the stone.

For special cleansing energies, you can add a very grounding stone like hematite. Use it like a second filter after the quartz crystal and imagine the energy moving through it as though it is a carbon filter straining out anything unwanted or draining.

For all of this you don't need a special or esoteric setting. Look for a suitable stone that appeals to you. Many people tend to think every agate is like any other and a rock crystal is simply a rock crystal. This is not true. They are like one family, but not every family member is the same. So, do a bit of soul-searching before buying a stone, focusing on whether the exemplar before you is a good one for using for your intended purpose.

Maybe you already have a good stone-fellow in your collection that would love to support you in your healing work. But if you want to use a new stone for this, carry it with you for a period of time and become familiar with it first. Try to feel if you would make a good team and take some time for it. No need to rush.

When people try to rush in spiritual matters they most often pay for it with later delays because things were not thought out. If you remember the old story of the tortoise and the hare you are on the right track.

If you feel that you would be a good team, speak with the stone about everything, and start to work together.

By the way, forget everything you've ever heard about "programming crystals." A stone is not a computer, and this is not all about "work," it's about a spiritual friendship. On occasion put your stones in the warm light of the sun, give them incense, or rinse them with cool water. After a while they will tell you what they want from you naturally, because it's important for the stone to cleanse its energy and regenerate, too.

If someone sees many patients each day, this ritual probably can't be done after every one of them. In this case it should be done in a concentrated form after the working day is through. As so often is the case, routine is key; when doing it on a regular basis, it becomes customary and works quite fast.

Of course, rituals like this can't balance out permanent overworking, as faced by so many doctors in hospitals, for example. We must be frank about that. They are made for the regeneration of one's own power, nothing more—but also nothing less.

Cleaning the Energy

As we are all different, not everyone is the kind of person who enjoys visualizations. There are many practical and hands-on approaches to help oneself, too. For example, some healers prefer to wear jewelry made from healing stones during their work and use it like a filter for the incoming energies of their patients. Tried and true stones for protection during healing are turquoise and hematite.

Necklaces and small body chains of healing stones can be used. Chains around the waist can help very much to "keep the energy together." In some African countries, waist beads, often made from colorful glass, are worn especially by women as more than just jewelry—to protect their personal energy field. In this spiritual area, embellishment and protection go hand in hand.

To put it briefly, protective jewelry should in some way enclose or encircle the core or trunk of the body (neck, chest, belly—at least one of them) and can optionally also be worn on the wrists or the ankles, as one prefers.

One thing also has to be mentioned here: it's not the end of the world if one has absorbed negative energies. This happens to us every day and is part of normal living. I want to place emphasis on that because some people live in constant fear of negativity. It's part of our life, and it won't harm us in the long run if we keep on cleansing in appropriate ways.

Spiritual baths have a long tradition for doing this job all over the world. There are some rules for it to work well. All baths are taken without any further bath additives (like soap, shower gel, bubble bath and so on). If you prefer to shower before the bath, go ahead, but the bath should be sacred, and one should take it in a calm and undisturbed atmosphere.

If you don't have a bathtub, don't worry. Make an infusion of the ingredients and once it's cooled enough, massage it all over your body for several minutes and shower it off afterward.

The Sage Bath

Pour one to two quarts of boiling water over a half cup of dried sage. Let it soak for about ten minutes. Strain it into the bathwater and enjoy for at least fifteen minutes. After the bath, dry off with a fresh towel and put on fresh clothes.

This one is an oldie but a goodie. Today many people look for things that are new and fancy. There's nothing wrong with that, but we should not make the mistake of throwing the baby out with the bathwater. Tradition is important, especially in our fast-changing world today, so hold on to it.

The Sea Salt Bath

This is also true for the sea salt bath. It's a classic and for a good reason; all life comes from the sea. The ocean is our big mother. All ancient myths reflect this. There's not one creation story without the power of the waters, and even science has confirmed that all living beings evolved from the ocean.

This is not just our metaphorical mother, and this bath is far more than just a cleansing bath (as it is often labeled). This bath means return-ing to the motherly source of life as we know it. It *is* about cleansing, but it's also about deep regeneration and renewal at this ancient source.

Use one cup pure sea salt for the bath, and proceed as stated above for the sage bath.

The Coconut Bath

This bath comes from African and Afro-Caribbean traditions, but Indian and Asian traditions also make much use of the coconut. All of them consider it to be a rejuvenating, cooling, and nourishing cleanser.

It's also a symbol of the head. If one faces stress—the kind of inner overheating that confuses the mind and makes one feel that they are not acting from their true self—then coconut is a good support, just as cooling of the mind benefits the body. Of course, the coconut is not native to European traditions, but this bath is simply too good to be left out and we can always be thankful when we are able to learn helpful things from others.

Put one to two cups of coconut milk into your bath. Alternatively, you can pour hot water over coconut flakes, let it brew for fifteen minutes, and strain it in the bath water. Coconut is a wonderful two-in-one cleanser, for it not only cleanses but also nourishes.

Mint Oil

The permeating scent of mint is a strong cleanser but also very refreshing for body and mind. It convenes the spirits of life in a person (the *Lebensgeister*, as we call them in German) and clears the mind.

It's quick to make: mix a few drops of essential mint oil into a carrier oil such as sunflower oil, almond oil, or jojoba oil. You can add more if you want more (for your temples against stress and headaches, for example). You can add less if it's for aromatherapy massage oil, which can help the whole body.

The rule of thumb is to start with a little. People's sensitivity toward essential oils is very different. Mint oil is a safe oil (but please don't use it on babies and small children), it's even edible, but when working with plants, more is not better—quite the opposite. If it's too much for you, your senses will be displeased instead of refreshed.

Spit It Out

Another method of cleansing that was practiced by healers quite often in the past is spitting after the patient had gone to prevent the jumping over of an illness. This way of cleansing was also used if someone had said something bad about a person, and it's also helpful against the evil eye (the powerful energy field of envy and malevolence that can hurt people).

Today this can be done discreetly by going to the bathroom. People working in a hectic hospital or who are very busy as healers can also do this while on break or after working hours.

Protecting Healthy Boundaries in General

Maybe you know the feeling of wavering boundaries. This can be the case if for example the moods and vibes of other people affect you as if they were your own, especially if it occurs with people you are not particularly close to. Taking things too much to heart is also a typical sign of weak boundaries.

But this can have many manifestations in real life. Some people tend to have a ravenous appetite for sweets, others drink too much coffee or get headaches or stiff necks. These are just some examples to show that this is not just a spiritual or emotional thing, it can affect the body as well. Observe yourself and listen to your inner voice—you know yourself best.

Our ancestors also knew about these problems and they loved to use red stones against this loss of power as well as for dealing with one's own life energy in a healthy way. Red corals and carnelians were especially popular for this. Red stones heighten one's vigor, give strength, and help to develop a good sense of self. Often people who need it the most shy away from the very thought ("oh, red is such a bold color, that doesn't fit me well") because they are so used to being exhausted by others. So, if you find yourself thinking that, think again.

If you decide to wear a red stone, it's best you use a chain or cord that is long enough to wear the stone over the solar plexus area. Some people experience feelings of being angry or churned up when starting to work with red stones. Nothing is without reason, there will be good reasons behind it, so it's good to investigate them.

If this happens to you and it's unpleasant for you (although a thunderstorm can clean the air at times), take off the stone, but stick with the issue it has brought up for you. Anger is never there for no reason, and ignoring it won't solve the problem. During your work with these feelings, wear the stone from time to time for a day to see how you progress. You can use it as a "mood thermometer."

When thinking about healthy boundaries it's also very inspiring to remember the healers of the past. Often they were real characters and off-the-wall originals. They had their principles in life and they stuck to them.

This is a huge difference to today, where many healing traditions try to be something for everyone. The old healers knew their possibilities but also their limitations and let no one walk all over them.

Besides the red stones, jet (also known as gagate) is highly recommended for people who face a lot of tension, as healers often do. In the old days jet was often used as a protection stone against the evil eye. But it also helps against envy, negative projections and burdensome tensions. It was customary to adorn it with a red bead (glass or stone) to make it even more powerful (more on this stone in the chapter about stones).

The Source of
Healing Energy

Not long ago I had to smile when I saw a woman indignantly complaining about a traditional healing spell book that had only Christian spells in it.

Well, what else did she expect? The vast majority of our European ancestors were Christian—at least in the time these spells were written, and of course this form of Christianity often differed a lot from what we understand by the term Christian faith today.

It was not without reason that up through the sixteenth century and even afterward, church decrees ordered clergymen to not perform magic and fortunetelling.

But we don't have to go that far in history. A while ago a woman told me the story of a pastor who was a friend of hers. One of his congregants had asked him to banish a negative energy from his home. The pastor was—to put it mildly—astonished at this request. But instead of explanations he was told by the congregants (who were clearly disappointed with the pastor's lacking abilities) that his predecessor had done this with the help of a black dog that lied down at the spot of disturbance. In this way, the negative energy was identified and thereafter banished.

This is pure folk magic, and the black dog exemplifies that the previous pastor knew what he was doing.

This shows how much magic is still there, just beneath the surface of modern rationalism even today. Of course, this applies not only to folk magic. Half of the country does "cosmic ordering" (author Bärbel Mohr's method has been very popular for some years here in Germany, and numerous books on it have been published in English as well), reads their horoscopes, speaks to angels in moments of despair, or lights a candle for a loved one in need—but absolutely no one believes in arcane things like magic!

How Does Healing Power Work?

We live in a time enamored with intellectualism, always trying to make things demonstrable and repeatable. This is difficult when it comes to magic. The true reason for this attitude is nothing less than a huge uncertainty. Plus we are trained to think this way from early childhood on, so it becomes our second nature.

The risk of this way of thinking is to lose the connection to the source that supplies us with power, not only for healing but also for life itself. A traditional healer who was also the head of a big Romany family analyzed this problem in words that can't be put better:

> Why do you try to understand everything? Leave the discoveries to those whose job it is to discover. Be content with what you are able to achieve, and embrace it.
>
> If you don't do this, all joy will escape from your heart through the hole of boredom and your hands will never again be suns for those with hearts and souls full of coldness.[6]

Or let's take Galsan Tschinag, a Mongolian shaman who studied in my hometown, Leipzig, during the German Democratic Repubic era. He knows both sides well, traditional and western, and said this about the westerners:

---

6. Derlon: *Heiler und Hexer*, 63

They are afraid. And critical, they doubt everything. I always call this the worms of doubt; the stuffed, brazen-unholy worms of mistrust. Many people consider this to be their strength. Doubt and mistrust are a culture, they think.

They always have a dark thought with them as their eternal shadow, which in the end always stands between them and the universe.[7]

Every spiritual healer who is true to himself and others knows that he does not know much at all. You have your spiritual path and your own thoughts about how healing works, but at the end of the day you don't know it for sure. The matter here is this: is this a question of knowing?

The first quote of this chapter hinted that discoveries are for discoverers, scientists, and scholars. This does not apply to intuition, feelings, and spiritual strength. While the rational approach suits many areas of life perfectly, we would be mistaken to think it would suit *every* area of life or that it's the only approach that is legitimate.

By the way, it's also true in science that the wrong approach won't lead anywhere, and a few scientists say that some of their major discoveries came to them in a dream or an intuitive moment.

Our rational mind is a wonderful tool to discover, classify, and rate things. But only the heart possesses the power that must flow for spiritual healing. This is also true for doctors, not only in alternative medicine. The classical doctor also has to reach the heart of his patient to make changes possible. For example, a doctor can tell a diabetes patient a lot of good reasons to engage in more exercise and eat a healthier diet, but if he does not get through to his patient on an emotional level, it won't click.

Of course, there can be many reasons for "clicks." It happens to smokers who quit from one day to the next. And not every patient wants to be reached emotionally and open up to the process of healing

---

7. Tschinag, 198

with all of its sometimes unsettling moments. Many just want a pre-scription for pills to fix it.

What is often overlooked is that an illness can become very famil-iar, like second nature to the person that has it. If this is the case, being liberated from that illness is like a shock to the system for the patient. Illnesses become like trusted friends for some and the liberation from it can feel very odd for someone used to this "friend"—a nasty friend, but a familiar one that often serves an (un)conscious purpose such as get-ting more attention, avoiding arduous things that otherwise would have to be done, etc.

You see, this topic is as complex as humans are. Healers, doctors, and non-medical practitioners can do whatever they can, but if the pa-tient won't even give it a try, they can't accomplish anything aside from just grabbing the prescription pad to provide some pills.

Of course, the not-wanting-to-change of many patients has deeper roots that grow from not-being-able. More than a few people are con-vinced they do not deserve healing. This brings us back to the topic of guilt that was already mentioned. Many people have a deeply archaic vision of illnesses being linked to guilt of some sort. The illness seems to be the penance for this guilt or wrong-doing.

These inner patterns often originate in childhood experiences ("This is because you were a no-good child!") and can be very deeply and firmly rooted. Most of these people are not even aware of it, so before anything else is done they have to be sensitized to think of themselves as being worthy of healing and that they don't have to "serve the sen-tence" beforehand.

But let's get back to the source of healing again. This topic is es-pecially important for traditional healers. For the prayer-healers of the past, this was a non-issue; they worked (and sometimes still work) with the Holy Trinity, Mother Mary, and the populous world of folk saints with their broad competences for almost anything (including even magic!). If you follow Christian traditions, you can find many books and websites dedicated to this topic. I won't be covering these saints in this book; not because of small-mindedness but because others simply know more about that area than I do.

For all those who would like to work with the old gods—I've listed them for you coming up! But please keep in mind that a personal connection to a divinity or entity comes above any list or description. If you can't warm toward an entity, any further effort will be useless. You have to be in tune with each other, otherwise there will be no true reply from the other side and it will be only superficial but not profound work.

If you find out that your favorite divinity is not credited for healing powers in ancient or traditional lore, don't give up too easily; simply give it a try. You can also cast and read oracles to find out more. Listen to your inner voice if there is a response from your divinity, or if there are signs in everyday life or in dreams.

What gods and goddesses are credited for in books and texts is just a small portion of what they *really* are. In the end all that matters is what happens between you and your spiritual team.

Healing Beings

The following list of healing beings is multicultural. I thought about this for a while: should I include only beings native to Germany or should I think globally? At first glance it seemed more consistent to include only beings from here. But what does "here" even mean?

Does the Egyptian goddess Isis count as "from here" or "from Germany" because she had sanctuaries in Mainz and Cologne, Germany? We can assume quite safely that she was not the only goddess or god feeling wanderlust and traveling throughout the ancient world.

Our ancestors were much more open-minded than many dogmatics today, and this might be the result of not yet reading all those wise books and, instead, learning from their own immediate experiences with the spiritual world.

What worked and what showed results spread. It's that simple. We tend to assume that our ancestors lived in a kind of ever-the-same "good old days." But this is not true; change has always been omnipresent.[8]

But what is especially important to me is that witchcraft is a *free* spiritual path. This means either you are free or you are not free. A little bit free is "the same as a little bit pregnant," as we say in Germany.

By the way, being free is not the same as being completely arbitrary. This is often confused or twisted on purpose to bad-mouth personal freedom and alienate free thinkers. Being free means that one is conscious about one's own decisions and sticks to them. What others think

---

8. See Parrinder for examples.

is not of importance. Another saying in Germany is if everybody sweeps in front of their own door, it's clean everywhere—meaning mind your own business.

It's not uncommon to find similar entities in different cultures; these are often called archetypes, the prefigurations of human experiences.

Let's illustrate this with a simple picture: look at an apple. In German it's an *Apfel*, in Portuguese it's a *maçã*, the French say *pomme*, the Turk *elma*, the Croats *jabuka*, and the Icelanders *epli*. But is the apple therefore in any way different or less apple-like across cultures?

Of course, there are still differences. Some cultures love apples and have many delicious recipes for this fruit; for others it's not that important. But the apple itself is always an apple, no matter if it's appreciated or not.

With spiritual energies, it's a similar situation. Different names were found for these energies or archetypes, but the power behind them remains the same. It's not so much about the name you call your "apple," as the core essence will always be the same.

When working with gods, spirits, and entities, trust first and foremost in your feelings and don't believe anything just because it was written down by someone, even this book! Remember: believing is not knowing. True knowledge is more than just understanding with the head. It comes from experience.

Never lose your sense of humor if you are uncertain or don't know which way to go. No pressure, no stress, please. Those two certainly don't help to get the healing energies flowing, so you're far better off without them.

Apollo

Apollo is the eternally youthful, golden sun god of Greek mythology and rules over the *arts* of healing like music and poetry. Today these arts are often not well known for having healing benefits. But some traditions seem to return; some Turkish hospitals have started playing old traditional healing songs for their patients after operations.

The effect of music is immediate. It goes from the senses to the emotions and into the body. Music can strengthen, calm, energize, or work your last nerve. Singing bowls can directly influence the body in this way, and waves of music not only flood the ears but also the entire body. No one would go to concerts if this wasn't the desired effect—to bathe in the music you love. And no one would feel well after a concert with music that is the opposite of their personal vibe and preferences.

Apollo is a good companion to work on anything that needs light and warmth. He's an expert for eyesight, clarity, and emotional sunlight. If you are uncertain who to work with, he's a good choice. The Hippocratic oath that doctors commit themselves to even now starts with him ("I swear by Apollo the Healer …").

When working with Apollo (also with other beings in general) you can create a small altar for him. In Apollo's case, cover it with a yellow cloth (you can also use paper napkins or a simple yellow bandana). Put a yellow candle on the altar and something that symbolizes your suffering, such as a bandage, a radiograph, a printed sheet with your laboratory values, a photo of the part of the body in question, or for emotional suffering, an abstract picture that you paint with colors and shapes that correspond with your feelings. Put some fresh yellow or white flowers, a piece of amber, and a snake symbol on the altar as well.

As soon as you have a quiet moment, light the candle and talk to Apollo, pray to him, or just meditate there. You don't have to "do" something all the time; sometimes it's enough to let the moment sink in, to experience a profound reinvigoration.

If this takes too much time and effort for your situation, just get a piece of amber. Using a needle or a multifunction rotary tool, if you have one, inscribe the name Apollo and the symbol of the sun, a circle with a point in the middle. Keep this stone with you. It's best to wear it directly on the skin.

Asclepius/Hermes

Asclepius is the son of Apollo, but in contrast to his radiant, beautiful father he is seen more as a down-to-earth entity. His birth was aided by

Hermes, and he learned the art of healing from Chiron and is known as an infallible healer, master surgeon, and wise herbalist.

In his ancient healing temples, temple sleep was practiced. This is an almost shamanic technique in which people came to sleep in Asclepius's temples to get instructions for their healing from dreams.

Today most of us would think: How can this work? How could they have been sure a dream would come? And what if it didn't?

Trust in our intuition is not very strong today. To understand, you would have to live in a culture where it's normal to go to a temple to get advice in dreams.

But still we can ask Asclepius for advice in dreams, in a half-asleep state, in meditations or in meaningful moments.

As with Apollo, the snake and laurel are sacred to Asclepius. One could view him as a half-human avatar of Apollo. As his birth was aided by Hermes, they are linked closely. They both have staffs with snakes as a symbol. Of course, they were not alone with this symbol, as Iris and the goddess of luck Felicitas also held the caduceus.

In some mystery schools Hermes is honored as a healing god because of this proximity to Asclepius. So, if you already have a connection to Hermes (or Mercury) you can also work with Asclepius in matters of healing. He is much more than just the messenger of the gods.

Baba Yaga

The word *Baba* means "grandmother" or "old one" in Russian. This ancient goddess is also known as Baba Yezi, Baba Roga, or Jezi Baba, and is a goddess of the woods, life, death, and rebirth, and in many ways is similar to the German Frau Holle (more on her a bit later). As is the case with many ancient goddesses, Baba Yaga can manifest as triple goddess or triad. In many fairytales and stories, she has two sisters, to whom she sends people that are seeking advice to complete various tasks as a test.

Even today Baba Yaga is a feared goddess. Even people with backgrounds in nature spirituality or Paganism tend to perpetuate the old stereotypes; they just express it a little more politically correct and call her a "dark goddess." But in doing so, they too continue to push the strong and self-determined female powers into the dark corner. Incorruptible female energy is still viewed as ambivalent, and simply calling her "dark" instead of "evil" is not a true shift in perspective.

Baba Yaga is known as an "old bone hag" because she accompanies people beyond death. She rules over the mythical water of life that resurrects people, an old analogy for the circle of rebirth.

We find in her an ancient shamanic goddess of waxing and waning. She has plenty of symbols, like rye grains, healing herbs of every kind, mortar and pestle, the broom, the poppy plant, the cauldron, the metal iron and of course Izbushka, her magical hut that stands on chicken legs and moves in a circle, as the sun circles around the earth.

Although many tales make her look like the stereotype of an evil witch, she can be very generous. For example, in Russian fairytales she sometimes gives inquirers a magical ball of wool that helps them find their way and make their fortune. There's no need to demonize her just because she likes to test the sincerity of people first.

In contrast with so many entities that were forgotten as time went by, Baba Yaga is still dearly beloved—despite or maybe precisely because of her gnarly appearance. (In Russian fairytale films she is often played by a man to illustrate her rugged nature.) She is a sly fox, a female trickster who helps people to reach their goal by putting them to the test.

If you want to work with her, I would suggest you first read some of her tales to get a feeling for her energy that bubbles up between the lines throughout. For a healing spell to invoke her strength, fill a mortar with a third of your favorite healing herbs, a third of rye grains, and a third of poppy seeds. Put a picture of the person in need into the mortar among the herbs and seeds. Cover it with the mixture and lay the pestle on top of it.

Light a white, a red, and a black candle (the colors of her horsemen who represent dawn, day, and night) in front of it and tell the old Baba about your healing wishes as well as what you (or the person in need) are willing to do for it. Let the candles burn down, and leave the mortar as it is until the condition of the person has improved.

Baba Yaga is especially helpful for serious problems and all female issues.

Bastet

Bastet, the Egyptian goddess of cats, is responsible for all things that make life worth living: music, scents, love, magic, dance, sensuality, and healing. Some records state that at her celebrations, similar to the story of Baubo and Demeter, the vulva was exposed, and laughter and wild dances took place to shake off all sadness and every evil.

Today Bastet is a wonderful helper when it comes to nervous problems, like tension and insomnia, and problems resulting from overworking or workplace stress.

Overworking is in itself a sign of a lack of joy of living, because one has forgotten that we don't live to work, but we work to make a living. This pattern often dates back to childhood experiences when accomplishments and "being good" (making the parents happy, proud, and so on) were more important than vitality and zest for life. It requires a lot of time and loving inner work to change this.

Bastet helps those who find it difficult to take care of themselves or who push others to take over the role of the care-taker and emotional nurturer. If you find yourself complaining "Because my partner (or child, parents, siblings, friend or whomever) behaves in a way I don't like, I can't be happy," it's high time for Bastet's joie de vivre. She brings you back to your own responsibility and helps to retrieve your inner power. Nobody is obligated to make you happy—nobody but yourself.

In my psychic work I sometimes meet people who wait years and sometimes even decades for a special person to at last behave "right," making them happy. This is very sad! They missed out on so many experiences all those years; so much joy passed them by. Not to mention the bitterness that arises if they realize one day that they waited in vain.

Wanting to be happy has nothing to do with selfishness. Rather, it makes you healthy and radiates out to others. Happiness "infects" others with confidence and courage to face life. People who claim that searching for more happiness is selfish are often envious or simply don't know how to find it for themselves and therefore feel compelled to put others off this ambition.

In this case Bastet is an affectionate teacher who helps melt the frozen soul, soften emotional hardening, and exchange grief for love of life.

To work with her, choose a Bastet statue or any cat representation you like. Photos and postcards are also a nice idea, the main thing being that it speaks to your heart. Give her perfume and incense, and play joyful music when talking to her, she loves music. Of course, in modern times she also loves to see (cat food) donations to animal shelters that give refuge to cats. Magic does not always have to be "magical" in the sense of candles, incense, spells, and all the like. It can also be done on a very practical basis.

Baubo

Baubo is the goddess of the vulva, which was sacred to many ancient cultures and a favorite symbol to ward off evil. She's the source, the origin, and the door to life. The divine vulva was often depicted in stylized form, like the diamond shape or the downward-pointing triangle. Cowrie shells also evoke this divine energy because of their form and were favored amulets in old Europe.

The motif of a goddess displaying her vulva is seen from the dawn of mankind. She even appears on medieval church walls as Sheela Na Gig.

In Greek mythology she is famous for cheering up Demeter when she was upset about the loss of her daughter. Of course, Baubo is also a wonderful companion during pregnancy and giving birth.

Baubo is an inimitable helper in times of crisis and despair, when things seem to lead nowhere and desperation abounds, for example during severe and/or long-term and chronic illnesses. She is a strong helper that brings back laughter. Her philosophy is don't wait until the rain is over for happiness. You'd better learn to dance in the rain. Although there is not a solution for everything, we are always in control of one thing: how we respond to the challenges of life.

You can awaken her power with a stylized picture or by wearing cowrie shells as jewelry. If you want to create an altar for her, use red candles and all shades of red that are pleasant to your eyes.

Red is the color of life and has been used since ancient times to ward off evil and illnesses. This is also true for the male version of this custom. In Italy people like to wear the *corno rosso* (red horn) to ward off evil. It looks like a small red chili pepper, a male phallic shape.

Brighid/Brigid of Kildare

Brighid is venerated as a goddess of divine light in witchcraft and has her holy day on February 1, also called Imbolc. Her special position is easy to see: she is venerated as a Christian saint as well as a Pagan goddess. Hers are the primal elements water and fire, but she is also a goddess of smithcraft, which links her to transformation and initiations.

She is especially helpful if you feel that an illness wants to say something to you, to discover its deeper meaning. Also, if complaints tend to recur and you can't figure out why you have this particular susceptibility, you can ask Brighid for the crucial spark of insight. She can be invoked for everything concerning healing, well-being, and self-awareness.

To work with Brighid in rituals, floating candles are a wonderful tool, for they combine her elements of water and fire. If you are not sure how to get in touch with her, go to a lake or river and meditate there, and this will give you the inspiration you need. If this is not possible due to your illness, have someone bring you a postcard with a lovely lake or river on it, visualize this place, and pray to Brighid to help you.

Cernunnos/Herne

Cernunnos is the Celtic god with deer antlers (his name, literally translated, is "the horned one") and it is very likely that his roots trace back far in history to the shamanic cultures of the dawn of mankind.

In today's spiritual work he helps us to calm down and ground ourselves. He is an elementary power and a wonderful helper if you don't know yourself anymore or when things get overwhelming or confusing.

If someone gets ill, some people show their true face and try with all their "good advice" to make the weakened person behave in the way they want. Such people are like energy vampires and don't really care for the need of the ill person; they just want to be seen as the glorious savior themselves rather than simply lending an ear. The vernacular puts it best, for "lending an ear" means to truly listen and not to talk about oneself all the time.

This is a very important point in general, so please keep it in mind when doing healing work or being there for someone who is ill. Sick people are often inundated with information, advice, and hints from others. But who listens to *them*?

Oftentimes all this handing out of advice is in fact a defensive behavior. I give you some hints, and while talking about all these helpful things I hope your pain won't get close to me.

We often tend to act this way, so it's really worthwhile to ponder that issue. Many people have so many obligations and duties during the day that they don't have the time and strength to really listen to someone in need. But one can feel very alone among the broad range of medical possibilities and therapeutic recommendations.

When your head is buzzing and you are insecure or perplexed, start meditating with Cernunnos. For this, take a statue or picture of him or a piece of stag antlers or stag fur; a photo of a stag will also do just fine. Light a candle at a calm place that you like and hold a silent dialogue with him. Ask him for support and to show you the right way—and ask him for the ability to recognize the right way. I learned this important detail from a woman who told me about her age-old prayer healer who always slipped in the phrase "and let me *recognize* the right way" into his prayers.

You can also ask Cernunnos to help you meet the right people at the right time or to make your social circle aware of the fact that you need more solicitousness now.

Also, it's good to think about compassion not as a one-way street. Ask yourself, "When did I last listen to someone in a quiet setting—just listening without giving advice?" Give it a try and you might be surprised how different and free the conversation will be if no one wants to be "helpful" and you are just there for the other person.

Cerridwen

Cerridwen is the goddess with the famous cauldron of growth and decay. Her holy animal is the sow (female swine), and this reminds us of Ceres and Demeter who also had this animal. Even Freya rode on a pig, indicating a similar cultural background: the goddess as nurturer, closely linked to the ground, where the ancestors are buried (and thus also linked to them).

There are many different aspects of Cerridwen and a book can only shine a light on some facets. Whenever you feel a god or goddess ring an inner bell in you, it's a good time to start to find out more. Try to find many different sources so you get a broad overview with many impressions.

Cerridwen is a nurturing healer; her energy often comes from food and of course she can be invoked for any problems concerning eating habits. A conscious and positive relationship to the food that nurtures us is her special domain. Her healing energy comes from the cauldron, and today this cauldron can take the form of pots, pans, baking dishes, and mugs.

Most hospitals serve their patients food that is tasteless and "cooked to death," which is difficult, because it's especially in these situations that we need good food. As an old German saying goes, good food keeps the body and soul together.

Many seem to feel this intuitively and so friends and family bring fruit, homemade meals, and so on to the hospital, even though the patients have full board there.

Elementals

The belief in elementals is found worldwide in different ways, but the root idea is very similar. In Europe we have four elements and they are linked to the spirits of fire, water, air, and earth. These elementals were often appeased to ensure good luck and given sacrificial goods to bring blessings.

A typical version of this is the sacrifice to the fire that is still common in many regions of eastern and southeastern Europe. For this, one gives a small portion of every food to the fire in the hearth. This is said to ensure the well-being of all family members. You could say a happy fire makes happy people.

The element air was often fed flour. Such sacrifices to the air were well-known until the 1960s in many parts of rural Germany. This shows that these customs were still alive not too long ago.

And even nowadays there is a German superstition that you always must sacrifice something to the water, so it won't take one itself (i.e., in drowning accidents).

Sacrifices to the earth were also very common, many things were buried in the earth to ensure a good harvest, and lucky tokens like horseshoes were put into walls of houses. Modern builders of their own homes will find many possibilities to do likewise.

Often the sacrifices for the elementals were food like cake, fruits, and grains, and the colors white, red, and black were included in the food offerings in some way. You will notice these colors often appear. They are symbolic of the beginning, climax, and decline of life.

Eshu

Exu, Legba, and Ellegua

During the time of slavery, Eshu travelled from West Africa to the Americas, and is now a global player—and player is just the right word here! Eshu is male as well as female and also everything in between, so I will be using "they" for a singular pronoun.

In traditional West African representations, they are depicted with breasts as well as a penis, one of their major symbols. In Brazil this evolved into Exu as the male part and Pomba Gira, his wife, as the female part. These spirits, with many different manifestations, live in the extensive realm which is often called Calunga.

Many cultures know beings of this sort, the divine tricksters in all their guises. They reign over the crossroads of life, making your life easy or arduous, and always appearing in some way unconventional and erratic. Many names have been lost, but their energy still shines through in the stories of Till Eulenspiegel, Robin Hood, and all the nameless jugglers and jesters of the past.

Entities of the crossroads are of course invoked most suitably at this place. If this is not possible (for example because you are bedridden or the crossroads within reach are too crowded and it would not be safe to go there in the quiet of the night) you can also use a photo of a cross-road, the crotch of a tree, or a cross.

In some traditions, crossroads in the shape of an X (where four paths converge) invoke the male energy while the Y shape (where three paths meet) invokes the female energy of this spirit.

Eshu can open or close doors in life. If you work with them for heal-ing, they can open the doors for healing to enter. Their colors are black and red, they love strong coffee, liquor, spicy food, sweets, honey, and strong cigars or cigarettes (if you can find a packet in red and/or black, even better). Their numbers are three and seven.

Just as many other independent and free-minded spirits, Eshu was often cast in a devilish light, but there is no devil in traditional African religions. She's the energy of chance. Everyone knows it well from life experience: sometimes you're up, sometimes you're down. We can lean against the wheel of life as much as we want to, but it will always be stronger than us.

Eshu can't be bribed; one can only ask for something, and it's always best to have a lot of humor, but then they are able to help in so many ways. They love to support the courageous, curious, and mischievous and will pester the self-pitying, furious, and egocentric. In other words: it's best to work with them if one can also laugh at oneself.

Fata Morgana, Fée Morgane, Morgan le Fay, Fairies

In German we say someone is *gefeit* if someone is immune to some-thing. The old diction of this word is *gefeyt* and there she is: the good fey/fairy that protects you and was known in the older Middle High German by the name *Feimorgan* or *Famuran*. *Fata* is the Latin word for fairy and, linguistically, fate itself (*fatum*) is very close to it. This puts a very different light on fairies than we are used to today, with all those cutesy glittery fairies, or the esoteric traditions that consider them only to be some kind of helpers at our beck and call.

Yet even today there persists the notion of the fairy that assigns the destiny of each child (often also in the form of three fairies) and who will one day stand at their deathbed to guide them back to the other side.

Women and men who are in league with these fairies will be great healers. But they are not allowed to cross destiny's plans. In many regions there are tales of healers who pitied the dying and turned their beds around when seeing the fairy approach (here we also find the motif of healers as clairvoyants, having second sight, and being able to see otherworldly beings). The ill person got well again, but the healer lost their ability to heal in that very moment because they flouted the laws of the fairies.

When I was a child those fairytales seemed to be very cruel to me. But there's an old truth in them: humans should not try to play god. We are not almighty, and the last word is up to the powers of life that we will never entirely be able to understand. We only see small details of the big picture.

Frau Holle (Mother Holle)

Precht, Bercht, Berchta, Eisenberta (Iron Berta),
Frau Gode (good woman), Hulda ("the well-disposed one")

Frau Holle is an ancient female goddess that is known by many names. As Eisenberta (Iron Berta) she has many characteristics in common with Baba Yaga, who also has a link to iron, being described in many tales with iron teeth or an iron nose, for example. Iron is a metal that is often attached to traditional shaman's clothing to subdue evil spirits.

As Berta, Precht, or Berchta, she is the lady of light, the white goddess (in Old High German *perath* meant bright, luminous and shiny). As Frau Holle and Hulda she is *hold* (meaning benevolent, kind, gracious) toward a person. And as Frau Gode, literally translated as "woman good," or more figuratively as "Mrs. Good," she is the good and benevolent woman, queen of the fairies and source of all life.

Frau Holle is a heavy hitter. She has many regional names which prove the vitality of her cult. She was never subjected to an *interpretatio romana*. (This was a common practice even during the times of witch trials in Europe. Many goddesses and "good women" had regional names that the women reported under torture. The Christian persecutors often did not write them down but summarized them as "Venus" or "Diana" in their case files, so the original and regional names of many other goddesses were lost.)

Her sacred plants are Wacholder (juniper) and Holunder (elder) and today more and more people are once again becoming aware of these sacred connections to be found in the names of plants.

Behind the fairytale figure of Lady Holle a mighty goddess of heaven and earth arises, being able to create the weather, ruling the seasons, and also healing, because she rules over growth and decay, waxing and waning.

Similar to Baba Yaga she comes for the dying to take them safely to the other world. But she also gives out little souls to women who wish to receive them as babies. She has a swarm of little souls around her and if a baby or child dies, it comes to her and is sheltered and cared for tenderly. She's a wonderful helper for all women and men who have sad and mournful experiences with unborn children in any capacity.

When working with her you can use her sacred plants elder and juniper, which both are invigorating and "reawaken the life forces" (revitalize), as we call it in German (*die Lebenskräfte wecken*). Rural folk as well as Travelers and Romany peoples especially loved the elder to cure many diseases.

You can take a white cloth and sweep it softly over the diseased area of the body, then tie it to an elder bush. Make a small sacrifice to the bush like a bit of honey, some milk, or three eggs (you can do as you please, these are just examples to give you a starting point), because one who expects help should give something for it, to maintain balance.

Freya

Freya is known to many as a love goddess, but as with so many "love goddesses," this is just one facet of her and it would be like clipping her mythical swan wings if one were to reduce her to a simple love goddess.

Her link to swans (often to hawks as well, but in our region the swans are prevalent) indicates that Freya is a goddess that travels between the worlds, a shamanic goddess, which were often linked with waterfowl. If it's difficult for you to travel to the land of Nod at night she will be a wonderful helper.

Besides the charming swan, she's also linked to the golden boar, a stout being that is associated with the power of the sun. His golden bristles are sometimes also seen as a symbol for golden grain. The boar is an animal of strength and this makes Freya not only a charming swan goddess but also a goddess of dynamic impulses. You are well taken care of by her if you suffer from a loss of joy and passion, or if your heart is heavy and you don't know how things could ever get better again.

Freya is also a great ally if you want to start a family, in all matters concerning pregnancy, birth, and taking care of little ones. She's also a great healer for the inner child in each of us. To connect with Freya's energies you might wear amber, her favorite gemstone.

Guardian Angel

Of course, the guardian angel can't be omitted in this list of helpful beings. Most people believe in guardian angels one way or another, no matter what their spiritual path is or if they even have one to speak of.

In ancient Egypt and Mesopotamia people already thought of angels as messengers between the divine and humans. Maybe this idea is as old as humanity; even the shamanic artworks of prehistory depict flying beings.

Angels are often seen as fundamentally genderless, but nonetheless some of them are seen as male or female, archangel Gabriel is often seen as a female being for example.

The guardian angel is a wonderful helper for healing work, especially for people with no special spiritual tradition. It does not feel like "some strange spiritual stuff" to them, because everyone is familiar with the expression, "You had a guardian angel watching over you!" when someone escapes a potentially dangerous situation.

In healing work it's most important that we mobilize the person's own inner healing powers, and this requires inner images and spiritual beings that appeal to the person emotionally and don't feel alien to them. There has to be some kind of connection there.

There are no rules on how to work with your guardian angel, because it's something that is very private and perceptions can differ a lot: some see angels as baroque putti, to others they are ethereal beings of light, and to some they are beings without any form as such, being pure energy that is sensed but not seen.

Stick to what is right for you. Not everyone is a visual person and people have many different perceptions—some feel, some see in their dreams, some see in their mind's eye—and the means of perception can also change.

You can arrange an angel altar with candles, flowers, fragrances, and a small bowl of water—water is a wonderful medium for spiritual energies.

Hekate

Hekate is a goddess of witchcraft and destiny and therefore also a goddess of healing, especially if an illness might determine the destiny of a person.

Today she is often referred to as a dark goddess, but we should keep in mind that her color in the ancient world was bright saffron.

It was Hekate who helped the desperate Demeter to find her daughter Persephone again. This story also gives us hints on how to work with Hekate in healing matters. She helps us to find the missing link, the unseen, that hinders us from recovery. She brings back our luck.

As a goddess of crossroads, she also holds the keys for all possibilities in her hands. This aspect of her has much in common with Eshu, who was already mentioned, as both watch over crossroads, the life path, and important decisions.

If you want to work with Hekate, create an altar for her in saffron with bright yellow candles (her traditional symbol of torches won't work well in a home, so candles are a good alternative). You can also go to a real crossroads to speak to the goddess directly.

Don't get too impressed with all the talk about her "darkness," and gain your own experiences. She's one of the most beloved goddesses of modern witches, and that would never be the case if she really was that grim fairy of gloom.

Isis

Isis is a healer par excellence. In mythology her special area of expertise is healing fragmented things that fell apart and now can't come together again easily. She has the power to give new life and is the goddess of life itself, always willing to provide a way no matter how bad things may look. Isis was called "smarter than the gods," and she is linked to the sea, the sky, the sun, the moon, magic, and wisdom. To bolster their reputations, the old pharaohs insisted they were her sons.

Many women feel drawn to Isis very naturally. Her power is strong, broad, and balanced and she's one of the goddesses who tend to respond quickly. Of course, this is a matter of personal experience, but in general some entities are more open, whereas others have to be pleaded with for a longer time or tend to be picky about whom they help (this doesn't so much have to do with sympathy in the human sense, it's more about the resonance of different energies).

Under Isis' protective wings (reminiscent of the protective cloak of many later Mary statues) you are safe, you can regain strength and arrange your life in new ways. If you are uncertain which entity you want to start with in your healing work, Isis is a wonderful choice.

Kobolds and House Spirits

In the old days one did not only address gods and goddesses for well-being and luck but also the good spirits, the "little people," or brownies that share our home with us. An undomesticated version of them is the garden gnome, and there is more to the good spirits than all the kitsch of little garden gnome statues. They are elementals of the earth.

In the home, these spirits had many names according to the region: little people, drak (dragon), or puck, coming from *pogge*, an old word for toad. This brings us to the ancient symbol of the toad as the source of life for the house, who was also linked to fertility and having children. It's no coincidence the stork was often depicted with a toad or frog in his beak.

Even in the present day there is a legend in many regions of a child that feeds the toad of the house with milk. The mother sees this, and, thinking that it's nonsense, she kills the toad. Soon after, the child dies.

These old stories are full of metaphors. If you kill the lucky spirit you also kill what makes you lucky.

This is similar to the stories of the white snake, also known as the snake with a golden crown. In legends she is the guardian of the thriving house and farm. If she was no longer appeased with a small bowl of milk because the young farmer thought this was nonsense, the luck of the house and farm would wane.

It's easy to work with house spirits. They love milk, honey, tea, and coffee and occasionally a glass of beer, wine, or schnapps. In healing matters they help a person bounce back. They give the house its blessing, but they can also withdraw it. If you face a sudden streak of bad luck, it's high time to remember them.

Mary

Mary, the "Christian goddess," has taken many older goddesses under her cloak. This often looks like the European version of syncretism and in fact Mary has adopted many symbols of older goddesses: the snake (most often under her feet, but it's still there), the crescent moon, fruits, lilies, roses, stars, dragons, trees, springs, and many more.

Mary had a tough time though; her role as mother of god was often debated in history, leading even to the assumption she could never have given birth to Jesus because a woman was such an inferior being. In medieval times many Mary-worshipping groups were prosecuted and punished as heretics.

The spearheads of the patriarchal church tried to diminish her wherever they could, but most people paid them no mind. They knew about and experienced Mary's help in their everyday lives. To this day in many German Catholic churches there are small plaques of gratitude next to the Mary statue, stating for everyone to see: *"Maria hat geholfen!"* (Mary has helped!)

In folk belief Mary is the merciful, understanding, and caring one. She helps, she soothes, and is there for everyone, no matter how hard it is. All the processions, the old traditions, the love and adoration for the divine mother speak volumes.

If your healing work tends more to the Christian ways you will find many places (many toponyms in German-speaking countries include "Maria" in some way and often indicate even older places of goddess worship), customs, traditions, and rituals you can work with.

But even if you follow a pre-Christian, Pagan, or polytheist path, you should not overlook Mary with prejudice. Many folk traditions and customs have preserved ancient goddess knowledge and passed it on to this day; this is where the syncretism comes into play. Look deeper and you will see that Mary hid many of her sister goddesses under her star-spangled cloak through the dark times.

Oshun (also: Oxum, Oehun)

Oshun is a goddess of rivers, lakes, and freshwater in general. A traditional phrase about her is she heals with her cool water. Today she is often typecast as a love goddess, but this is just half of the truth, as we have already seen with Freya.

Let's have a closer look at the symbolism of water, because another traditional saying about her is "no one is an enemy to water." And how could one be, because this would mean being your own enemy. Water is life, from the smallest cell to the biggest organism: nothing would happen without water.

In healing, Oshun helps to cool down external afflictions. Inwardly she makes the juices of life flow again and helps us to dissolve what is stuck in the body, mind, and soul.

Oshun can be met at rivers, lakes, and streams, but especially at waterfalls and cascades and in warm summer rains.

She loves cinnamon, basil and honey, which has to be tasted before being served to her. Her number is five and her colors are white, yellow, gold and amber.

These are some of her traditional correspondences but always keep in mind your personal experiences, too. What is received in personal work with a being always takes priority.

Sara (la) Kali

Literally translated as "black Sara," Sara-la-Kali or Sara Kali is the matron saint of Travelers and the Romany people. She's one of the famous black Madonnas and her shrine is in the small southern French village Saintes-Maries-de-la-Mer. The traditional pilgrimage to her takes place in May.

Sara Kali is often invoked for healing, but she can do a lot of things. Some people trace the origin of the Roma back to India, and it might be that this Romany saint has an ancient link to the Indian goddess Kali, as they are quite similar and Romany people are said to have their roots in India.

In everyday life Sara Kali is often invoked for healing because of her balancing power. She protects people who got into difficulties through no fault of their own, and she protects people during travels. This is also to be seen figuratively: if an illness is a journey (not a nice one, but with the positive destination of recovery) you can handle it in a very different way. It helps not to think "this has to go away fast, or better yet, *very* fast," but instead to think of the illness as a path that has to be traveled; the symptoms are the key for healing.

Of course, this can't be applied to all kinds of illnesses. If someone has a heart attack or a stroke, every second counts. But if you have time don't rush too much. Many things are treated over-hastily or in the wrong way, because one is impatient and feels urged to do something. We get squirrely over things that our grandparents would have seen as: "Hold your horses! First let's have a good look at it."

If you feel this urge, if you feel helpless or don't know how to go on, if you haven't (yet) a clear diagnosis and everything seems to be vague, Sara Kali is a wonderful help. She helps to find the right and possible way to reach your goal and to feel better.

Triple Goddesses

Matrons, Fates, Urme, Norns, Goddesses, Moirae, Fati, Muhmen (Aunts), the Beths, Schicksalsfrauen (women of fate), and others

Triple women (sometimes seen as goddesses, sometimes more like a kind of fairy) go by many names. In Celto-Roman areas they were carved on sacred stones and known as the Matrons.

Some people think that the triple goddess is a modern invention of Wicca and similar ways, but it's much older and has just been reawakened today. For example, Hecate never really got lost and was often depicted as a triple goddess on copperplate engravings of early modern times. There are also the three spinstresses of the traditional German fairytale who help the young heroine of the story to succeed (helping her spin the thread of life). And, of course, not to be forgotten are the three witches of Macbeth.

Sometimes these triple women reflect the classical roles of the three fates: one brings luck, one is rather neutral, and one brings the misfortune a person is to experience during life. The Roma of Transylvania had the Urme, who could be either good or bad and often appeared in groups of three—some sources translate Urme as "fate fairies." Such a trio were the Norns as well: Urd (spinning the thread of life), Verdandi (measuring it), and Skuld (cutting it). The names can vary a lot between different regions, but the roles are always the same. These three divine women reign over the destiny of humans, their lifespan, their luck and misfortune.

The grouping of three women appears in Christianity as well; the three Marys are especially well known. There are also the three Beths (a

German group of virgin saints: Einbeth, Wilbeth, and Worbeth) as well as the three holy maidens, Barbara, Catherine, and Margaret.

They were often invoked in matters of health—both for humans and animals, to "turn" bad luck and to see happier days.

To this day, they are wonderful allies in healing matters. You can make an altar for them by putting three female symbols (such as shells, female dolls, bowls, cowrie shells, ribbons, stones, or whatever inspires you), a bowl of water, and a candle on it. Feel free to decorate and arrange it until you feel it to be harmonious.

Yemaya

Iemoja, Yemowo, Mami Wata, Janaína, La Sirène, Yemalla

Yemaya has many names and different lines of traditions, but one thing is for sure: no matter what name you call her, if you do it with love and respect, she will answer.

Yemaya is the mother of the sea, the source of life. She's also the sea we are from, the amniotic fluid. Her sacred colors are blue, silver, and white, her number is seven and among her symbols are the sun, the moon, stars, and all maritime things, such as the wheel, anchor, boats, fish, pearls, and shells. In some syncretic traditions she is very close to Isis.

You can come to Yemaya with any concern, she's "big momma" par excellence, soothing, healing, and encouraging. It's not possible to ascribe one special area of healing to her, because could there be any suffering a real mom would not care about when her children come to her?

She likes to help with emotional issues and everything concerning children (including the desire for a child) and family in general (as well as dark family topics and things surrounded by a veil of silence). If you feel desolate, lonely, and forsaken, if you are sad or have problems with emotional closeness and trust (and if it's difficult to find out whom you can trust), request her help.

She likes to show up in dreams and meditations, but also while half-asleep or daydreaming, which is a favorable time for communication between spiritual worlds in general.

So how to choose the right helper? Well, we have a saying in Germany that might be helpful for that: the first thought is the best. This saying proves to be true time and again. The first thought is pure; it´s free of pondering and over-analyzing. It´s the spontaneous spark of intuition answering the question at hand.

Follow this initial spark and stay open. It´s not uncommon to be handed over from one spiritual being to the next during the journey to healing. They are all experts in their own ways and when you´ve mastered one step it might be that another being "adopts" you for the next.

Sometimes this reminds me of a teacher-pupil relationship. One energy teaches you what you have to learn and afterward you are turned over to your next lesson with another teacher. So this is not so much about choosing a particular being, but more about spirited relationships.

The Right Time

It's always fascinating to see that common things like the names of the weekdays, which most people never would think about, can tell us so much about history and the intellectual world of our ancestors.

Of course, we live our lives in the modern day. It would make no sense to transfer old traditions into our time unaltered. Nevertheless, knowledge of the old ways can be a great resource, especially in our fast-paced world that is constantly breaking up old rules and structures. Which is in itself not bad and gives us more freedom, but it also tends to overburden the individual.

Living in tune with the knowledge about the old days of the week and the moon keeps one grounded. Moon calendars have recently become very popular again in many households (and it's not just people interested in spirituality who are buying them).

Some old calendars are centuries old, like the German *Steinhausers Kempter Kalender*, an old traditional folk calendar, which has been printed continuously since 1692. It's similar to *The Old Farmer's Almanac* in the US, which has been printed since 1792.

Many people say, "Well, I don't stick to it meticulously, but I like to plan with it because it gives things a natural order." And why not? Moon calendars help us slow down and give back a healthy feeling for the natural cycles of life.

The Days of the Week in Traditional Folk Magic

The old lore of the days of the week still clearly shows a mixture of Greco-Roman, Celto-Germanic, and Christian traditions. In the fourth century the Germanic peoples adopted the Roman week, and the energy of the Romans gods, linked with the days of the week (as we will see in a moment), still echoes in rural and folklore traditions.

Monday

Monday is linked to the moon and its energies. As the moon phases change constantly, the day of the moon is also seen as a changeable day and it's better not to start new things on this day. As the old German saying goes, "Monday beginnings—no good proceedings."

Another saying is that what you start on Monday "won't grow old"— in other words, it won't last. This knowledge is common to this day. In Germany, if a particular device is full of bugs and doesn't work properly we call it a "Monday model," and it's been proven that the error rate at work is actually higher on Mondays, resulting from the break of the weekend, as our bodies and minds need their time to readjust to working mode again.

The old traditions state that on a Monday you should not lend money, wear new clothes for the first time, bake, send the children to school for the first time, cut your hair or nails, or create or sign contracts. You should also avoid starting a trip or moving into a new home, and for heaven's sake you should not marry on that day! Everything that can wait one more day should be left to rest on Mondays.

For healing work this special day has its advantages, though. It's not the best day for things that you want to develop with stability, but it's very helpful if one hopes for a change. This means that everything that is intended to initiate a shift of the current situation can be done on this day. If changes have come to a halt, if things are at a standstill, then Monday is a great day to give it a nudge.

Tuesday

Tuesday is the day of Mars in the Roman week. Old traditions say that everything which is better avoided on Mondays can be done on a Tuesday, because heaven smiles on new endeavors on this day. Whether one plans to marry, to start a new business or to move in a new home, Tuesday is a great day for all new beginnings.

In the old days Tuesday was also a favorable day for taking a healing bath (with herbs and essences) because this day quickens and revives the body. But with one restriction: "warlike" or aggressive interventions to the body—things like operations—would best be avoided, if possible.

Tuesday is a very good day for magic meant to strengthen or bring an initial energy boost. It's a favorable day for all spiritual healing work. While Mondays have a hazy and gently mutable energy, Tuesday is more like banging a fist on the table.

Wednesday

Wednesday is the day of Mercury and, like the moon, he is seen as a vague energy; because Mercury is so flexible, it can turn in any direction. So, Wednesday is also not a good day for things meant to last but a very good day for things to *change*, and this should be mirrored in the direction your healing work takes. It is similar to Monday, but Wednesday is male (or androgynous) and has a more bustling energy due to the connection to Mercury.

In old traditions Mercury reigns over the nerves, so one should take care to avoid overwork and stress that would result in headaches on this day, and in general steer clear of stress and never overwork. Rather, Wednesdays are wonderful days to strengthen the nerves with meditations, relaxation exercises, or aromatherapy massages. Everything that brings you back to your center is favorable, and scents and herbs are especially beneficial on this day.

Thursday

Thursday is the lucky day of the week, ruled by jovial Jupiter and outshined only by Sunday. Medicines are thought to be doubly effective if taken on a Thursday.

Strength and health are multiplied through everything one does on this day. It is also a good day for healing baths and seen as a wonderful day for detoxing, since Jupiter is astro-medically linked to the liver.

This is also found in old hints that one should never fertilize (or spread manure) on Thursdays; it's a day of clearing out, not of absorption.

If that seems contradictory, that's just the nature of folk traditions. The general sense of Thursday is that it is a day of metabolism. Some people interpret it in the negative sense (don't fertilize) while others in the positive sense (medicines are doubly effective). Both approaches co-exist.

Friday

Friday is Venus' day and everything relating to the skin and beauty is very favorable on that day. But as with Monday and Wednesday, one should not start big and important things on this day.

But in contrast to Monday and Wednesday, it is a very good day to get married and to play the lottery or gamble, because Venus is the "small luck" in classical astrology (and Jupiter is the "big luck").

Venus's day is also very good for cartomancy and predicting the future. Roots for healing magic were often dug on Fridays or Sundays.

The changeable energy of Venus can also be used to "turn" illnesses for the better (more about that in the section on old healing methods). This was done by conjuring up the climax of an illness to abate it from there on.

This day is also good to go to the hairdresser and cut your nails. (In the old faith it was important to cut the nails if one wanted to get rid of an illness, so that only healthy things would grow from then on. The nails were burned or buried under a tree.)

Since the rise of Christianity this day is fifty-fifty a lucky and an unlucky day. Lucky because of the goddess Freya (giving it the name *Fri*-day or *Frei*-tag as we have it in German). Unlucky because of the Christian Good Friday. In folk belief, even in modern times, it is a day that evokes mixed feelings depending on the perspective: the enchanting Freya or the day of suffering of Christ in the later religion.

Of course, the day of the fertile goddess was a favorite to sow and plant. This can also be an interesting aspect for healing work: invoking creative energies and preparing a fertile ground.

Saturday

Saturday, it's not difficult to guess, is the day of Saturn and very favorable for long-term and chronic matters and our bodily structure in general (bones, teeth, ligaments, joints). In the old days this was the preferred day to do cupping and blood-letting.

Today we often appreciate gentler methods: detoxing tea, for example, with nettle and horsetail is very beneficial on this day. Visiting a sauna or steam bath is also a very good idea on this day.

Saturday is called *Sonnabend* in some regions of Germany, meaning "evening of the sun" or "Sunday eve" and the evening of this day was especially holy. This has a link to the old Celto-Germanic custom, when the new day started at dusk and not at dawn, as we know it today. On Saturday evenings it was forbidden to work, because the Sunday day of rest already applied to it.

In German we have two words for this day, showing how history comes into play even with things as ordinary as names for the days of the week. Besides *Sonnabend* there is also the word *Samstag* for this day, coming from the Old High German word *sambztac* which was introduced during Christian proselytization along the Danube River. So, to this day in western and southern Germany the word *Samstag* is used most often and in north and eastern Germany the old Germanic *Sonnabend* is used more often. In Low German along the coast it's called *Saterdag* (quite close to the English Saturday, isn't it?), and there we have a clear link to Saturn.

Sunday

Even nowadays Sunday is the holiest and luckiest day of the week. Sunday's children are seen as especially lucky people because they are close to the spirit world. Unfortunately, many clinics today tend to induce labor on weekdays because of financial reasons (Sunday premium pay) so far fewer children are born on this lucky day.

But a glimpse into history is interesting here, too. Until the thirteenth century, the lucky Sunday's children were Saturday children, because the

Jewish Sabbat was the lucky day of the week. These Saturday children were seen as natural spirit seers and were consulted when inexplicable things happened (in some Eastern European regions this custom is still alive). The link between Sunday and lucky children came later when the belief in spirits was diminished. Depending on the region, spirit seers were much-respected advisors and healers, but in some regions they were also feared and had to live a life on the edge of society.

Sunday is the best day for healing work, but it has to be done in a relaxed manner. Sunday is the day of sacred rest in the old traditions. People who've just recovered from an illness should not be active on Sundays, but rest until Monday before resuming work and daily duties.

It brings bad luck to be in a rush of hustle and bustle on this day. These old rules of luck and misfortune were often wise guidelines to avoid pathogenic stress. Clothes sewn on Sundays were said to bring illnesses, but we can't translate this old custom literally to today, because in the old days sewing was work while today (for most) it's a relaxing hobby. One was also not supposed to cut trees, fingernails, hooves, or plants on Sunday. Humans, animals, or plants—everything was seen holistically in those days.

Today we should see these old rules as inspiration, and maybe bring back the good old Sunday walk through the park or nature again. Many people are a little tense on Sundays because, as we say in German, "they stand with one leg already in the work week to come." Our wise ancestors knew better: because, as we have seen, they didn't start anything important on Mondays anyway, it was a much gentler start into the new week.

One more thing: Sunday was a very good day for a wedding, for that's not work but a celebration.

Please Keep in Mind

When it comes to weekdays and the choice of fortunate days in general, it's important to use common sense, too. An important operation or an urgent treatment should never be rescheduled or delayed just because of the day of the week, the moon phase, or other things. Life is influenced by many factors, not only the moon or the day.

I am adamant about this because blind superstition is not helpful. In my work as a spiritual consultant I've heard many stories of people shifting important treatments, for example because their astrologer was against it—and who suffered damage because of it.

Please always keep in mind: it's good to know and apply the old knowledge, but it should never be misused carelessly or as a substitute for common sense.

The Phases of the Moon

The fundamental rules about the moon phases are easy and many will know them already. If the moon is waning you treat things that should vanish, minimize, and disappear, like warts for example. If the moon is waxing, it's a good time to strengthen the body and to nourish it.

The new moon (meaning the dark moon, not the new crescent) is a good time to start new things and initiate positive changes.

This is the view most of us have today, but you can also go by the old rule of new moon: a day that is taboo for any magical work. This wasn't meant as negative, as we tend to perceive these limiting rules today. It was simply a day of "moon rest" in the old days. So even the good old moon had a day for privacy and quiet—when it could rejuvenate, so to speak.

The full moon, on the other hand, is the moment of maximum strength and can be used for any kind of luck and blessings. But folk magic often prefers to work in the days prior to that (usually one to three days before full moon) so the energy is still rising and "pulls up" the magic with its increasing energy.

Besides the waxing and waning of the moon, the signs of the zodiac were also of interest in folk magic healing. Please keep in mind here, too: urgent treatments should never be delayed because of the moon. Today some folks tend to overstate these old rules in unhealthy ways, but even the old healers taught that the moon can facilitate many things, but in times of upheaval you have to do what has to be done.

Following the path of the moon through the zodiac is very easy: the zodiac starts with Aries, which is linked to the head and so it goes on step by step—or rather sign by sign—down the body. Certain signs, such as Taurus with its ruling planet Venus, also have additional meanings. So, Taurus is not just the neck but also (typically Venus) especially good for skin and beauty matters.

The Signs of the Zodiac and the Planets

In the following list I refer to traditional astrology, as our ancestors used it. In matters of healing this is also useful because the "new" planets Uranus, Neptune, and Pluto are so-called transpersonal planets, meaning that they influence the fate of whole generations. This section will examine the moon's journey through the zodiac signs and their respective planets.

Aries and Mars

Aries rules the head and everything concerning it, like headaches, migraines, and the brain, as well as everything that can affect the head, like sinusitis. The ruler of Aries, Mars, is associated with the blood and traditional "blood cleansing" (today it's called detox), but also can be used to improve blood circulation.

Mars is the planet of power and when in Aries this gets heightened further. So, if one suffers from listlessness and a lack of vigor, the days of Aries should be used for spiritual work.

Taurus and Venus

The areas Taurus rules are the neck and the throat. As it was said above, its ruler Venus also makes it a wonderful day for beauty treatments of any kind. Since Taurus is an earth sign, applications of healing earth, rhassoul (Moroccan clay), or mudpacks are especially effective. You can take this link to earth literally in your healing work.

Gemini and Mercury

Gemini rules the arms, the shoulders and the lungs (as these come in pairs). Since Mercury is the ruler of this sign it is also linked to the nervous system and troubles like restlessness, jitteriness, and insomnia. Try reducing your coffee input on Gemini days (when the moon passes through Gemini); you are already alert on these days and too much might overshoot the mark. As an air sign, Gemini doesn't tend to calm down Mercury's high-flying energy. But if you are in need of some good brainstorming, these are your days!

Cancer and the Moon

Cancer rules over the stomach, gallbladder, spleen, and liver—all innards between the lungs and intestine and bladder, to put it simply. The Moon also adds a link to all things feminine, like fertility, the female cycle, and hormonal balance. So, everything concerning these topics is also very fortunate on these days (especially if the moon is waxing).

Leo and the Sun

Heart and circulation are the main healing areas of Leo energy. If one wants to alleviate troubles in this area it's also important to remember one's own Leo lion-strength and move, work out, and take life into one's own hands again.

Many illnesses of the heart and circulation have their roots in unhealthy food, not enough exercise, and a constant lack of time coupled with stress. The lion—and in small form cats, too—are wonderful reminders of being the queen or king in one's own realm and making a new set of priorities.

As a male sign of the Sun, Leo also supports any kind of men's health issues, as Cancer does for the women.

Virgo and Mercury

Virgo supervises digestion, which includes the bowels and all metabolic processes that are linked to them. Virgo's planetary ruler Mercury links it to the nervous system as well, and while this may be surprising at first glance, our ancestors already knew what science is just beginning to discover: the bowel has an entire nervous system of its own, the enteric nervous system. The "gut feeling" is not just proverbial, it is very real and is sometimes called our "second brain." Sometimes we make decisions based on gut reactions, with our brain in the belly.

Libra and Venus

Libra rules over the kidneys, the bladder, and (just like Taurus, who's also a Venus sign) everything concerning beauty and attraction.

If we look at attraction and beauty not in a superficial way, but in a deeper sense, we see that they have to do something with harmony. It's all about coming to terms with yourself and respecting your own unique balance. And what could be more appropriate for this as a symbol than the two scales of Libra?

Scorpio and Mars

Scorpio is the sign of the sexual organs, and, due to his ruler Mars, is also linked to strong elemental powers. As we already saw with Aries, this is about blood, the life force itself, and the energy that makes life continue.

Mars is not just about fighting, and this is often overlooked. He's also about vitality, vigor and assertiveness.

Sagittarius and Jupiter

Sagittarius is the sign of the upper leg and its veins. Its planetary ruler Jupiter also links this sign to the liver and the muscles. This makes Sagittarius days especially effective when it comes to sports, workouts, or just a good long walk in fresh air outside, to refresh and rejuvenate.

Capricorn and Saturn

Capricorn is an important sign in the old moon traditions because it rules the knees, skin, bones, and joints. This comes from rigid Saturn, being the ruler of everything firm, supporting, and defined (like the skin that encompasses the body).

Because Saturn is linked to the earth element and also attributed to cold, warming applications are especially good on these days and it's also important to wear warm clothing so as not to catch a chill.

Aquarius and Saturn

Aquarius rules the lower leg and the veins in it. Contrary to Capricorn, Aquarius does not link the Saturn energy with more of the earth element, but with the element of air, and this combination is much easier, not so stiff.

Aquarius days are the best for working with chronic ailments of any kind, because Saturn represents stability and the element of air brings changing energies, or the proverbial fresh air, into it.

Pisces and Jupiter

Pisces rules the feet and is especially good for reflexology and our inner grounding in general. Also—as with Sagittarius—Jupiter brings the areas of musculature and detox (the liver) into play.

But where Sagittarius (being a fire sign) is more about the dynamic and sporty aspect, Pisces as a water sign tends more to the emotional side of life.

Psychosomatic problems can be addressed especially well on Pisces days. And psychosomatic does not mean imaginary, a common misconception. It means that it's rooted in the soul, but the illness itself is manifest.

It's also a good day to help find solutions for unclear problems, where the reason has not been found yet.

Because Pisces is the last sign of the zodiac, it was (and is) traditionally used to get rid of things and to banish them before the next moon cycle through the zodiac begins. Many still know that this is especially effective to get rid of warts, but you can adapt this for any problem you want to banish.

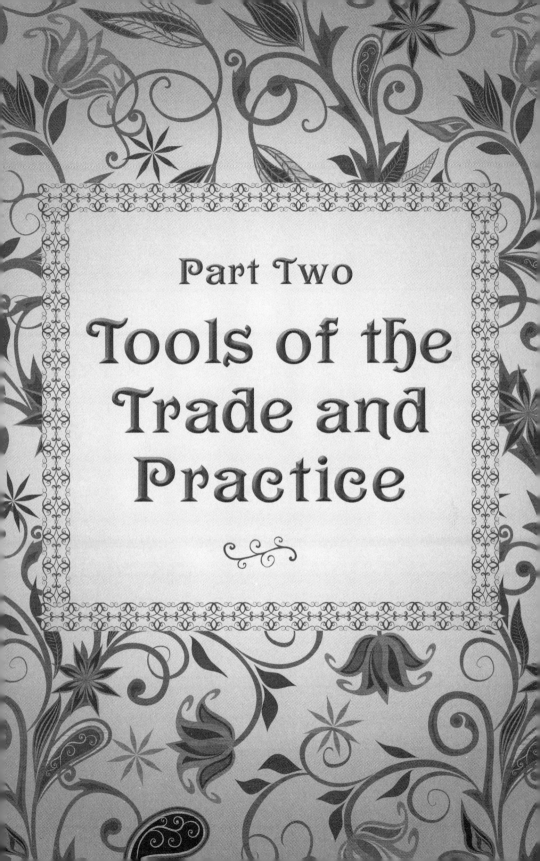

Part Two

Tools of the Trade and Practice

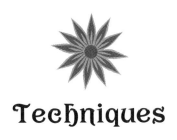

Techniques

The long list of spiritual healing methods passed down from our ancestors cannot be easily catalogued, in part because different regions and healers prefer to utilize or combine a variety of techniques. No wonder—we are talking about a living healing practice as opposed to a recorded one. The terminology can also be confusing. Terms vary and occasionally we find a discrepancy in terms applied to one and the same practice. This is important to keep in mind when dealing with the old techniques.

Good healers consider each patient as a unique individual. Even when they present with the same symptoms, healers will treat a forceful, dynamic person differently than they would a meditative or melancholy person.

We can only approximate the traditional healing methods in this book. In practice they are a thing of intuition and experience. In general, healing can never be learned from books, although they serve as good advisors that no experienced family of healers cares to do without. Spiritual healing is something that is constantly renewed and changing the moment the healer connects with the patient.

Blowing

Blowing means just that: the healer blows on the ailing part of the body, much like we still do with children today when they get hurt. Traditionally the blowing should be in the pattern of a cross three times. As a side note, we still use the German expression to "make three crosses" to express relief or gratitude when certain events do (or do not) happen—as in, I'll make three crosses when this is over! These crosses, when blown on the body, do not necessarily symbolize the Christian religion, but were seen as signs of protection in the old folk beliefs. Some healers also use this blowing of cross patterns after a treatment to seal in the work and to help the patient hold on to the newly acquired strength.

Böten/Blessing/Praying Off

Several regional euphemisms exist for the German word *böten*. They all have the recitation of a phrase, saying, or blessing in common. These spells are part of the healing practice. They can be murmured, spoken in thought or written down and carried on the body. As with all healing techniques that include the spoken word, it is important *how* these spells are spoken. One cannot be hesitant, but must utter the spell as you would a deep truth that rests within you. It does not matter whether you do so in thought or out loud. It should in no way sound fearful or pleading; nor should it sound overly authoritative, which belies insecurity too, after all, or you wouldn't have to start out so drastically. Speak your words calmly as though you were uttering an unwavering truth. I often picture a deep, dark blue mountain lake in my mind's eye. Not necessarily the lake itself, but the feeling that such a lake and color evokes.

Find pictures like that for yourself. You do not need to see them, but can feel them or remember a certain smell or a sound. The method is not important as long you conjure up a strong "true" feeling. We will refer back to mental images in the later section on magical spells.

Drawing Through

As with wiping off, drawing through includes getting rid of an illness through motion. People used either old standing stones for this purpose, drawing the sick person through them, or split a tree and pulled the patient through the gap this created. The tree was later carefully tied together and sealed, so it could continue growing.

Drawing through is rarely practiced today, mainly because it is hard to find an arrangement of large stones that would offer a place for the practice. The method itself was widespread. It can be traced back deep into Eastern Europe.

Hoops present an alternative to the method. They are magically decorated and crafted and finally swept across the body and the person steps through them. Wooden hoops like the ones children use for hoop rolling and hula hooping are best used for this practice. They can also serve as the basis for an herbal wreath to be braided around the hoop before the person steps through it.

Egg Applications

Eggs play a preeminent role in folk medicine when it comes to absorbing illnesses and drawing them out of the body. Certain numbers held symbolic significance here (nine was a common number for eggs). The healer would use these eggs to roll across the body of the patient from head to toe, slowly and with deep concentration. Afterward the eggs were either buried or sunk in the river.

This method can be found in many regions in the world. It can also be used in self-care. This means that one rubs the egg across the affected body part, carries it out of the house and —as mentioned—buries it or throws it in the river.

Eggs are excellent tools in regard to spiritual cleansing as well. They are a symbol of life and hold the power to take on and neutralize extremely negative vibrations.

Exercise, Source of Strength, and Relaxation

As you may have noticed, I did not use the word sport, but exercise. The body wants to be exercised. This is twice as true for people whose occupations demand that they sit.

In today's world we often associate exercise with spending money. People are convinced that only the purchase of a fitness video, a gym membership, or special clothing will effectively lead to physical well-being.

This is not true, of course. Exercise has always been free. What matters is that you do something; it makes much more sense to spend ten minutes dancing around the house to loud music a few times a week than to purchase a yearlong gym membership and never go.

You should also forget all the overblown regulations and dogmas that surround health and fitness. We're told that exercise only takes effect after thirty minutes and we have to completely exert ourselves. If you get the chance, talk to someone in the exercise sciences. I spoke to a professional and was told that studies exist that oppose pretty much any principle telling us how to "best" exercise. What matters is simply what works for the person who exercises. We are all unique individuals and this needs to be respected. After all, our goal is not to become professional athletes, so why all the pressure?

Isn't it better to say that *any* form of exercise counts? That makes the whole enterprise motivating and fun. Don't compare yourself to others, even though that is sometimes hard to do. There will always be someone who is fitter, more agile, or more light-footed than you. Then again, there are also those who can only dream about moving as gracefully as you can. I learned something in the three months I dealt with my knee problem and was forced to spend the majority of my time sitting down: exercise is precious. Being able to move is a gift. Sometimes you truly don't know what you have until it is gone. I found myself bawling at times, because the uncertainty about what was going on with my leg and the inability to walk (in the most beautiful spring and summer seasons, no less) made me feel angry and helpless at the same time.

The body needs time to make changes. That means what we call laziness, in our tendency to have huge expectations, is much more reasonable in most cases than charging ahead with too much steam only to receive the payback in the end. Let others thrash about. That's their problem. Find exercise routines that fit you personally: beautiful walks, dancing, swimming perhaps. Be gentle with yourself and take pleasure in it. If you can still enjoy it, you're in a good space. By enjoyment I don't mean the arrogant smile that some people use when boasting about their latest impressive feat at the gym, but a delicate flow, a good mood, and gentleness. It's not a contest. Have the ability to recognize when enough is enough.

You will still need your body for a little while, so be good to it. We are talking about the golden medium: muscles and joints want to be in motion and exercise is important for the soul and spiritual equilibrium. Think movement and joy instead of overdoing it.

Be careful to choose something that is fun for you, because if you don't, you will do it two or three times at the most or (even worse) you will go through with it, but get no enjoyment from it. Enjoyment ensures that you will do it on your own volition without the need to talk yourself into it with clever arguments. The weaker self the fitness industry tries to persuade us to believe in with its "holy-be-that-which-makes-you-firm" mentality does not exist. What does exist is the wrong form of exercise: that which is not enjoyable and causes you to deceive yourself. You will know when you have found the right method for you when you look forward to it as the highlight of your day instead of viewing it as a chore.

The positive effects of exercise cannot be measured, but must be experienced. One day I discovered that my persistent sleep troubles had disappeared. I suddenly found myself falling asleep at night without problems. It dawned on me: could this beneficial rest be a result of the fact that I started swimming? Was it really that simple? Can a body that is not physically challenged keep you awake because it retains too much energy? Even though I was mentally exhausted at the end of the day, maybe my body remained wide-awake because it was not challenged enough.

Exercise adds something positive to the entire organism, not just part of it. Everything is connected within the body. We can't treat a problem in complete isolation. We have a choice to view this in two ways: "Oh, how horrible … my problem affects even the parts that were healthy" or "how wonderful that the parts of me that are healthy can contribute to balancing out the part that is not."

Forget the popular image of the perfect human form that the world of fitness particularly likes to focus on. We are all crooked and off-kilter in one way or another. A completely "correct" human being does not exist. We would be praised with a "naturally grown" label if we were apples. We are a product of nature and as such are better compared to an apple than a Barbie doll.

Laying on of Hands

The laying on of hands requires that the hands be held above or directly on the body. Healing energy is then sent from the healer to the patient.

Hands have a special symbolic significance. Drawings of hands appear even in the earliest cave drawings of mankind. Amulets in the form of hands are said to repel negative energy and meant to protect the wearer from evil.

The laying on of hands carries a further significance, since a lot of people live their daily lives with little human touch, if we discount handshakes or gestures of that nature. They have nothing to do with deliberate and gentle touch, meaning healing touch. Touch can have a deep-reaching effect on one's emotional life, as any physical therapist will tell you. Occasionally people can start crying in the middle of the healing session because the massage loosened knots in the tissue that retaining a certain emotion.

Most people experience a feeling of warmth or a subtle tingling sensation during the laying on of hands. It is an extremely personal form of healing and as such can have deep-reaching effects: literally hand-ling the patient in every sense of the word.

Again, it is important to pay close attention. If you are determined to consult an expert in this practice, be sure to go to a healer you trust; ask other clients about the healer, do some research to make sure you feel comfortable. More than one woman has told me that she experienced the "laying on of hands" as a sexual assault. These women then fled the situation in haste in the best-case scenario. If you can't find a local healer you trust, there is certainly nothing wrong with experimenting on your own, with your partner or with close friends. It's a thousand times better to do "amateur healing" yourself than to go to a "powerful" healer that is misusing his or her position.

Please always remember: Where there is light there is shadow and the desire to be healed should never override a healthy dose of common sense or lead to situations that are not good for you and potentially even dangerous. If you are unsure, consider bringing a person you trust to the healing session with you.

Light, Air, and Sun

In addition to magical remedies, our ancestors also considered light, air, and sun to be holy remedies in terms of driving away diseases. My old family doctor—she was well into her seventies even then—used to prescribe at least a half hour walk in the sunshine for any number of ailments. Her standard sentence was: "Go outside for half an hour every day—I don't want to hear excuses. Sunlight has an effect even on cloudy days!"

Comfortable beings that we are, we often think, "If only that were so easy." But it *is* so easy. Everything else simply has to do with our treasured comforts. If we consider how many hours people spend in front of the television when they claim to have no time, it becomes clear that in reality it is a matter of not *wanting* to do it instead of not being *able* to do it.

I remember well how my grandmother would drag me out into the fresh air on day three of a cold (at the latest), regardless of whether or not there was snow on the ground. No excuse was permitted. I was bundled up and off we went. "Child, you have to get out into fresh air or you won't get well!" was Oma's enduring pronouncement.

. What can I say? She was right! Our walks never failed to give me new strength and I quickly became healthy again, even though I did not always feel like walking at that particular moment.

Moving in fresh air is one of the best fortifiers—and bonus: it's free. If we believe the chrono-biologists and anyone in occupational medicine, we know that lack of light is a problem that leads to listlessness and lack of energy.

So many people spend all day in enclosed spaces and instinctively feel that this is not really good for them. In the winter we often hear this sentence: "I won't see the sun all day now," if the sun is not yet up on the drive to work and the ride home is again spent in darkness. I can only recommend what our ancestors already considered holy: Spend time in fresh air every day, even if it is only for five minutes. That is better than nothing, after all.

Pegging or Plugging

Pegging again utilizes trees as healing helpers. It is an ancient, tried-and-true healing method. It involves drilling a small hole into a tree and filling it with a piece of cloth that holds the disease symbolically. The hole is then sealed with a peg.

Most people would have a hard time boring into a tree in this fashion today. We have a different relationship with trees now. Nevertheless, I would still recommend this method as spiritual support in severe cases. After all, the motivation would not stem from disrespect, but true psychological strain. The hole does not have to be big or deep and if you should happen to find a knothole, you can use that as well.

Turning

Turning is a generic term for all practices that serve to bring an illness to its turning point: the moment at which the patient's self-healing skills begin to gain the upper hand. How this was achieved was fairly ruthless at times. Traditional shamans still like to cause brief moments of shock when it comes to mobilizing their patients' healing powers and to break through blockages. These are the proverbial healing shocks. In everyday life, for instance, we assume that scaring someone will cure hiccups. In fact, most of the time that does work.

Research has shown that the composition of our genes can be measurably influenced. Is it coincidence that shamans so often describe their work as the re-ordering of a new body and soul?

Of course, a strong stimulus to turn an illness can also be triggered in a positive way. A cold can be wonderfully turned in children by symbolically locking it into a bottle and throwing it away. By having fun with it you can not only re-strengthen their healing powers, but also restore a feeling of "I'm the boss around here." Healing has a lot to do with self-confidence, as well as faith in both the strength of your own body and your ability to take good care of it.

Tying or Fastening

Traditionally, ailments were tied to a healthy, strong tree, preferably on a Thursday or Sunday, at sunset during a waning moon. While I am happy to share the specific timing preferred by our ancestors, this method can of course be individually adapted today. We do not live in the times of our ancestors and they do not live in ours. We cannot always adhere to the old traditions in their original form, although it would be a shame to see the old ways disappear entirely.

First, brush the sickened part of the body with a cloth or a ribbon or string, which is then tied to the tree. The tree, being the big, strong living organism that it is, is supposed to absorb and neutralize the illness.

We encounter exceptions here, too—occasionally people chose trees stricken in years, whose frailty and possible fall symbolized the passing of the illness. In this case use the healing magic with the old analogy "Just as this [tree] fades, so the illness shall fade." In general, I would suggest the use of big, strong trees bursting with vitality.

Visualization

Our ancestors did not use big words like "visualization," but many healers used mental images and their imagination in their work. They went inward to see things.

This way of thinking is hard for us today. We (too often) separate and sub-classify the holistic stream of perception in dream and daytime consciousness—both our inner perception and outer concepts. We make it way too hard for ourselves.

We will deal with healing spells in the following chapter. These spells repeatedly conjure up concrete images that relate to healing. Many healers speak of light or dark, and sometimes different colors that they perceive in their work. They purposely conjure up certain pictures throughout the healing process.

Wiping Off and Removing

During the practice of wiping off and removing, or brushing, or sweeping away, the ailing part of the body is symbolically wiped or brushed off (either a few centimeters above the skin or with skin contact). The illness is thereby wiped away as if sweeping the body to cleanse it.

The healer most often shakes his hands after each stroke or after the completed treatment to shed the negative energy. Some wash their hands in cold water afterward.

Strokes are performed away from the body and generally top to bottom or—a wide variety of possibilities exists here as well—radiating out from the heart.

The old healing formula of "wipe it off, heal it off" stems from this technique and can be thought or spoken aloud when performing the healing practice.

Today methods like this would be referred to as aura massage, aura brushing, or something similar. However, these methods were known in our area long before the hippie movement and the Indian influences that came with it.

Sometimes tools or aids were applied; in these cases, the sweeping was literal, and a person was swept off with a broom or a brush instead of hands (if a broom was used, the person was first covered with a sheet to protect the skin). This broom treatment also came into practice whenever an illness was traced back to the evil eye or a curse.

Sweeping can be wonderful as a preventative method. Brush massages with the appropriate visualization can be used to sweep everything negative or evil out of one's personal energy field.

Writing Off

Magical healing phrases, blessing phrases, and occasional combinations of letters were written onto a small piece of paper. The piece of paper was then folded up and carried on the person or in clothing. Sometimes the paper was even swallowed like medicine. This is the process of writing off ailments and can still be used today with old phrases, affirmations, wishes, and symbolic lettering.

In the old days, people did not use just pieces of paper, they also utilized metal plates, stone, wood, or pastry. In some traditions healers used gingerbread in particular. A magical formula was carved into the gingerbread and it was then fed to the patient in small pieces until the entire gingerbread was consumed.

Magic Spells
and the Power of Words

Before I begin: I am repeating all spells in the exact form in which I have received them from my sources. I have made no changes.[9]

Of course, I understand that my readers follow a variety of spiritual paths. That is why I want to make one thing clear: anyone can make changes to the spells and add the spiritual powers to which they feel connected. It does not matter if you prefer to work with Jesus, Mary, the great goddess, Cernunnos, Isis, your spirit animal, or angels. Just do it. The possibilities are endless.

We can approach this the way our ancestors did. They spoke to the powers they considered holy. A change like this will not weaken the spell, but make it more powerful than one involving a force that holds a negative connotation for you. You can come up with your own spells, as well. We will discuss this later on.

The terminology for the use of magic spells and prayers can vary greatly depending on the region. A friend who grew up in Bavaria had never heard of the term *böten*, yet he was familiar with the concept of praying off from his own childhood. However, even though the terminology may differ from region to region, the overall structure of the spells remains surprisingly similar regardless of their region of origin.

---

9. In this book spells are no longer printed in their original languages but in an English translation. Some of the spells rhyme in German; whenever possible, the translation has been adjusted so that the English will also rhyme, but only when it does not change the literal meaning of the spell.

We tend to underestimate the power of the word. We endlessly talk and type and are practically surrounded by clouds of words in our daily routines. It is not always easy to find our way back to the origins of the power of the word from here. Our ancestors considered words to be a central force in the healing process. It was important to use meaningful, symbolic, and magical words instead of small talk from everyday life.

I was originally doubtful when I began dealing with magic spells in *böten*. I thought about all those people looking for the perfect spell to perform love magic. A spell that can change reality by the simple sequence of its words, regardless of the circumstances. We all know that the bare sequence of words has no effect unless we infuse them with energy. If they are spoken with love, however, the old (or new) healing spells hold great powers.

We can only speculate why that is. Perhaps we dive into an ancient healing current when we apply them.

We have learned to believe in miracles, but in some cases, we need incredibly dramatic examples: the painless operations performed with kitchen silverware by Brazilian trance healers or the operations executed with bare hands we have seen in Asia. When we witness things like this we can put our skepticism aside for a moment and find ourselves in awe of the miracles that can happen when we are not so scientifically minded that we declare them impossible. Is it possible that we are sick with arrogance, with coolness, with our because-nothing-can-be-that-may-not-be attitude? How small our inner world is—yet we believe ourselves to be so incredibly advanced.

The old healing spells have nothing to prove. They are simply there and weave words and healing energies into a powerful combination. The following spell from ancient times leaves a great impression of how strongly our ancestors believed in the power of words:

My word is big,
My spell is powerful.
My word is stronger than water,
Higher than the mountain,

More desirable than gold,
More powerful than a rich man.
My spell cannot be disturbed by water,
Nor by fire,
Nor by the earth,
Nor by the air.
He who drinks all the water from the sea,
Who rips all the grass out of the field,
Even he can't overwhelm my spell.[10]

The mention of the four elements and the comparison to nature is reminiscent of old shamanic incantations. The choice of words leaves the impression that the spell holds deep magical powers that transcend mere words alone.

Do we have the self-confidence to speak spells like this today? This is another important point to consider: commitment and determination are important components when it comes to healing with spells. Don't leave a back door open for contingency plans, but commit to what you are doing wholeheartedly. The magical spells used in praying off, *böten*, turning, and talking off were often considered blessings in order to differentiate between them and everyday speech.

These spells were all invented at one time or another. Some are very old, some relatively young. In the past as well as today, many healers created their own spells, tailored to their experiences or by spontaneous inspiration.

If you are out to create your own, keep it short. A four-lined stanza or a short symbolic tale is ideal.

Not every healer uses spells. Some simply have an inner dialogue with God, Mother Nature or an angel to achieve the healing. The spell does not necessarily have to be in the strict form of a rhyme.

---

10. Hampp, 23

Perhaps you ask yourself why the mental pictures conjured up in these spells are so important when the healers often murmured them quietly or simply repeated them to themselves.

It is essential that the people who heal have a picture in their mind's eye that they can project onto the person who is seeking help. The words serve as a path to the mental picture. It is not always about the words themselves, but about what they convey. They always carry a picture or a story, which is supposed to have a symbolic effect on the ailment.

The powers of healing tales appear in all cultures even today. Fundamentally, the magic spells of our ancestors were no different. Even though the healing tales sometimes only appeared in the form of a four-lined stanza, they always conjured up an image.

The spells were generally repeated three times (in serious cases even three times three times, so nine times; or three spells were used in three sessions). This was then followed by a gesture: blowing three times in the pattern of a cross, for example, or stroking the affected area in the pattern of a cross, sometimes drawing a cross with an index finger or a thumb in the air above the area. Be careful to ensure that the lines of the cross point away from the patient, not toward them.

After people learned to read, spells were traditionally passed along on pieces of paper. It was the job of the designated successor of a healer to record them while the healer dictated.

To make a spell your own, it is helpful to copy it by hand in order to acquire it mentally.

Healers were not of one opinion on whether or not it was allowed to pass on the spells. Some were adamant that the spells needed to remain a secret in order to retain their healing powers, while others passed them along because they felt that there were so many people who were suffering. You have to decide for yourself how you prefer to keep the tradition.

Dear readers, I would like to ask you to use the spells freely, but with respect. They should not be uttered unless there is a reason to do so.

If you would like to learn them by heart, only repeat them to yourself mentally. Don't turn it into a show when you apply the spells or pose as a great healer or anything of the sort. Ultimately, greater powers than humans are at work in the healing process. Healing work and personal vanity do not mix well.

Have faith in the spells. Do not think to yourself: what if it doesn't work? It is not up to you whether or not it works, anyway (we are neither God nor the great Goddess, after all). So, do your best, do it with love, and without hesitation.

The old healers stressed over and over that they were not the ones doing the healing, but relied on the powers above. This attitude is psychologically helpful because it prevents us from freezing up from fear of failure and disgrace in the event that it does not work. This sensation of freezing or cramping up is exactly the reason why the whole thing would not work as well as it should.

It is possible to apply the spells in self-help situations, although not all healers do this. It used to be common sense; who would sit around and wait with painful burns if they know a spell against burns, for example?

Spells for Afflictions

The following spells are classic *böten* blessings. They can be found in countless traditions with subtle variations depending on the vernacular and the personal interpretations that people added.

I can't cite the source of the well-known spells because they are considered common property among healers. I am citing spells that I found in single sources or received from individual healers, of course.

Many blessings are still popular today. Some were even turned into folk songs like the famous *"Heal, heal, little goose."* Mothers still hum it over wounds of their children today:

> *Heal, heal, little goose;*
> *Everything will be all right soon.*
> *The kitten has a little tail;*
> *Everything will be alright soon.*
> *Heal, heal, bacon from a mouse;*
> *In a hundred years it will all be gone.*

Interestingly enough, bacon plays an important role in several magical instructions. It is supposed to be applied to the affected area and later buried at a crossroads, under a tree, or in a cemetery to banish the illness.

We can only guess that the use of bacon was originally part of the spell. It is not unlikely, since the spells often referred to an ingredient that was applied during the recitation.

This spell works in a similar fashion:

> *Healing, healing blessing*
> *Three days of rain*
> *Three days of snow*
> *Nothing hurts anymore!*

We still blow on a wound if a child falls down or has any kind of injury today. As soon as they are familiar with this ritual, the little ones let us know unambiguously: "You have to blow on it!"

That's what I call an ancient healing practice transported into today's times with no problem.

Atrophy

Atrophy in folk medicine refers to all illnesses in which people experience significant weight loss or a general weakness. The following spell serves to strengthen a person and can be combined with other spells.

> *Gain in the limbs*
> *Gain in the flesh!*
> *Gain in the veins and the blood*
> *As certain as the moon shines in the sky!*

This spell was preferably spoken during a waxing moon. It only makes sense then, because the moon functions as a visible symbol for the desired increase (in strength, vigor, weight, etc.).

Bladder Infections

Mother Nature knows quite a few remedies for bladder infections. Tea made from stinging nettles can effectively treat the first signs of an infection in most cases before it gets a chance to truly nest. Healing methods involving spells were familiar with this problem as well. The following Northern German spell proves it:

Cutting water and travelling water each turns off with the other.[11]

The term "cutting water" refers to the ailment. Travelling most likely refers to a flowing body of water.

Our ancestors often included their natural environment into the healing magic. As a result, it is more than likely that this spell was spoken next to a flowing stream while the affected person relieved themselves.

Blood Blessing

(to stop bleeding and heal wounds)

Naturally we go to our doctor when we bleed or have large wounds in order to get them wrapped. I note these spells primarily for traditional reasons. They can be useful on your way to the doctor or (in case of larger injuries) while waiting for the ambulance to arrive.

Some traditional healers can stop the flow of blood in the blink of an eye and heal wounds without leaving the trace of a scar. Don't forget, they have a lot of experience with this. Therefore, do not perform experiments in serious situations! Common sense is always the best counsel, especially when it comes to healing work.

> *Lord Jesus walked through the alley*
> *Where blood and water flowed.*
> *He let the water flow;*
> *He stanched the bleeding.*[12]

---

11. Schmidt, 103
12. *Lommersdorfer Chronik*, 193

Another saying is:

Moses walked through the Red Sea.
He struck the flood with his staff,
And still it stood,
And so shall you stand, blood.

The motif of Moses splitting the Red Sea can be found in many old blood blessings. It is a pious image that served our ancestors well in the treatment of bleedings. The "Red Sea" was not meant to be parted, but assuaged.

Three oak trees stand in the green forest.
Under the oak trees sit three spinners.
One runs,
The other licks,
The third stands still.[13]

This blessing is reminiscent of the three Norns as spinners of fate. It is unusual because it cannot be traced to Christian roots but seems to originate directly from a much older time.

Three blissful hours have come upon this world. In the first hour the Lord was born, in the second hour the Lord died, in the third hour the Lord was resurrected. I now call these three blissful hours and quiet you, N.N.[14], and so still the blood and the fluid in your limbs. I thus heal the injuries and wounds to them.

Many variations and embellishments exist for this Christian spell. Its core serves to transmit the resurrection of the sacrificed Son of God into healing the patient.

---

13. Hampp, 42. Note: the licking here could refer to when women wetted their fingers when spinning to keep their work running smoothly.

14. N.N. indicates the name of the afflicted individual.

Those who follow the Christian path can keep the motif of the crucified God. You are free to change it to similar mythological figures like Wode (Odin, known under this name especially in northern German healing spells), Dionysus, Persephone, Inanna, Veles, Ishtar, Xango, Shiva, or Osiris, depending on your personal beliefs. In ancient mythology both Gods and Goddesses undertake quests to the underworld. It is not restricted to male deities.

Among blood blessings we can't forget the tried-and-true Longinus blessing; it dates back to the time between 945 and 1000 CE:

> *The knight Longinus was the man,*
> *who saw the wound in our dear Lord Jesus Christ.*
> *The wounds bleed a lot,*
> *Stanch blood through the holy honor.*

Longinus was the legend of a soldier who wounded Jesus on the cross, stabbing him in his side with a lance. The blood he drew supposedly healed his blindness. He was then baptized and preached the Gospel. Be that as it may, the blessing was never lost and is still being used today, a clear sign that it has been proven effective.

Burns

In folk medicine, burns (or "fire") refer to all infected or inflamed skin conditions, burns, sunburns, erysipelas, and fever. This includes illnesses that naturally have heat associated with them, which can also include allergies. Allergies are generally an "overheating" reaction of the body to often completely harmless stimuli in the environment.

In certain cases, ergotism (St. Anthony's fire) was also included in the term burns. It posed a serious health threat in the old days. I am including it as a historical annotation.

I will refer back to rashes known as "the rose" later, since it had a special place in healing spells. However, spells against burns can also be applied to the rose. In folk medicine it is considered a subcategory of burns.

Burns, fall into the sand,
Fall into the path of the wheels,
Fall entirely away.
I stanch this burn[15] and throw it into the sand.

It is common practice to sweep across the affected area with a cloth (the material does not have to touch the skin) and bury it afterward.

This blessing is my personal favorite. It once saved me an afternoon by the lake, among other things. I had just bought a piece of cake and a freshly brewed cup of coffee at the kiosk when the paper cup slipped out of my hand as I was sitting down. The hot coffee spread so thoroughly across my leg that the thick denim material instantly soaked it up. The pain made me drop the cake from my other hand. My first thought was: my skin will blister from the heat! My second thought was (this happens in a fraction of a second in a situation like this) about the Swabian women who get the spells in their family as a spiritual first aid kit at weddings. They were not highly regarded bringers of healing, but ordinary women, so let's try this!

I said the burn spell quietly to myself and drew three little crosses across the area with my index finger. The pain stopped instantly. Only a short tingling sensation and the leg felt as if nothing happened. When I checked to see what the area looked like under my pants I could not even find a reddening. The leg looked exactly the same as the other.

I am writing this story to encourage all those who believe that only great healers and highly praised masters can have an effect. I am no healer, and was not given mysterious initiations. I am merely an author doing research on the subject to preserve the old knowledge. I acted without worrying about whether or not it would work. I simply had the strong wish that it would. I would have looked for a doctor without hesitation in the event that it did not work and heat blisters had developed. I would like to stress this: it is not about turning off practical thinking, but if the solution can be this easy, we'll gladly accept it.

---

15. Or: *I take this burn.*

The rhyme in German, *Brand auf Sand* (burns on sand) can be found in many spells against "hot" ailments. Sometimes the burns fall into the sand, sometimes it is tossed into it. It can also sink into it or many other options. Next to the obvious rhyming advantage, this also paints an effective picture because sand absorbs heat well. It soaks it up. Since "burns on sand" doesn't rhyme in English, you may choose to modify these spells to "burns on earth" for the assonance of the phrase (e.g. "burns, fall into the earth"), as the earth cools and absorbs heat just as well as sand does. Rhyming, alliteration, and other poetic devices were often used in spells to make them sound better when repeated, and thus more powerful when spoken.

Here is another blessing for burns:

Go away from us burn and not into us, whether you are warm or cold, stop the burning. May God protect you, N.N., your flesh, your blood, your marrow, your limbs, and your veins. May they be safe from the cold and warm burn and go unharmed.

This spell calls on God for help (as with all spells you are free to change the deity depending on which powers are best to bring healing for you). At the same time, it invokes healing for the entire body. It is not simply about the affected area, but the body is holistically treated as a complete system. Mentioning the name of the sick person (N.N.) strengthens the magic.

The second part of the spell from "May God protect you ..." can be used separately to strengthen someone in convalescence after an illness. Simply replace the words "from the cold and warm burn" with "from illness." You can also add it to the end of other spells, if the body is supposed to be strengthened overall in addition to the affliction that is addressed.

Spell-based healing was and is a creative art. It is not about copying. Feel free to add your own personalization.

Three holy women are doing the wash.One beats,
One rinses,
The third puts out the fire.

Here we again meet the three holy women who populate so many healing blessings. The picture of washing as it is portrayed in this blessing makes sense and the ending "puts out the fire" makes it clear how this blessing works. It utilizes the magical principal of opposites: water fights fire and takes its power.

St. Lawrence sat on the glowing gridiron.
God came to him with comfort.
With his strong, almighty hand,
He extinguishes the cold and hot burns.

St. Lawrence appears in many burning spells on account of his martyrdom by fire.

In doing this we stay faithful to magical thinking; like heals like. If a holy person has experience with fire, they will also be able to help with burns on the mortal plane. In some spells the holy person is the one who heals, in others—as in the example above—God himself appears as the helper. As God stands by the holy person, he is supposed to stand by the afflicted and take the suffering away.

Mary once traversed the land
And found a red silken band.
She picked up the red silken band,
And so healed the red spread.

Mary and the saints have a lot of wanderlust in these old spells. They enjoy walking the land. This is a promise: they are near; they will come by and help you. The activities that they perform are symbolic of the healing of the illness. As always, our ancestors spoke in pictures, because they knew that healing happens on the basis of mental pictures and a spell isn't much good unless it evokes an inner picture.

> *I warn you of ninety-nine types of fire.*
> *One builds the fire,*
> *The other splits the wood,*
> *The third blows on and off.*[16]

The third line in the text is especially significant since it can be assumed that blowing occurs during this spell, meaning that people would blow on the afflicted area three times in the pattern of a cross to banish suffering.

If more than one helper is involved, they always show up in threes:

> *In the early morning dew,*
> *Three beautiful virgins were walking.*
> *One walked through the green grass,*
> *One searched for the leaf of a lily,*
> *The third took the fire.*[17]

Cool dew and fresh vegetation function as pictorial means of healing to conquer the burn.

The three beautiful women are part of a long tradition. They are anchored in the cult of the three matrons, which is reminiscent of the three Norns. There were many sanctuaries of holy women in Germany and these are documented through findings of altars and hallowed stones. It is assumed that they are of Roman-Celtic-German origin. However, it is likely that these figures can be historically traced back to

---

16. Frischbier, 49

17. Hampp, 52

much older times. (See "Triple Goddesses" in the Healing Beings chapter.)

Spells against burns can be extremely helpful in everyday use against minor burns (grease spray from a pan, an iron, etc.). Therefore, it is good to learn at least one of them by heart.

It usually takes a little bit of time before a spell takes effect. You should simply try it out. Don't make a big deal about it, but simply murmur the spell three times with calm concentration over the affected area. Next, draw three crosses over it with your index finger or blow three times in the pattern of a cross and see what happens.

Cancer

We are all aware that we should discuss this disease with the utmost care. I do not want to give anyone false hope.

Nevertheless, I have decided to include the following spell because it can instill new courage to accompany medical treatments. Even when it comes to cancer, a person's spirit plays an important part in recovery (as with any illness).

We do not wish to persuade anyone to neglect medical treatments. However, if this old spell allows just one person to gain new confidence, it will have done a lot of good.

So go into the deep red sea.
There is a table and dish.
On it lays a baked fish.
Eat and forget human flesh and blood,
you don't do any poor human good.[18]

The analogy of this spell is simple: it offers a tasty meal to the illness—in this case baked fish—instead of allowing it to devour the person. The illness is supposed to forget its current "favorite meal,"

18. Hampp, 98

meaning the sick person. This spell can also be used with all other illnesses that threaten to hollow out a human being.

Colds and Fevers

Spells against burns generally work for fevers as well, since it falls into
the category of a "hot" illness as mentioned above. Still, there are a few
spells that can be applied to fever directly:

> *Fever, Fever!*
> *I'm telling you: Leave me!*
> *Go, shake gray stones!*
> *Go, shake tree trunks in the forest!*

When we ask the fever to enter into gray stones, we are reminded
of the burn entering into sand. In this spell, the heat is banished to both
stones and tree trunks.

Trees often play the role of a mighty plant in healing spells. In comparison to us relatively small humans, trees can cope with illness better
due to their size and strength. We can transmit illnesses to the tree to
neutralize them.

> *Cough, go away!*
> *You, cough of N.N., do not scratch the body of N.N.!*
> *Cough, go away!*
> *You, cough of N.N., do not scratch the bones of N.N.!*
> *You, cough of N.N., do not scratch the heart of N.N.!*
> *Go along the sea,*
> *Scratch the stones of the sea,*
> *Scratch the sand of the sea!*
> *They taste better than the body of N.N.![19]*

This spell is another good example of thinking in picture form.
This is an integral piece of magical spell healing: The scratch of the

---

19. Both spells: Hamp, 99

cough becomes the center of the spell and the cough is addressed as you would address a person with whom you can negotiate. This is a deeply shamanic way of thinking.

The illness is not aggressively banished in this spell, but rather we appeal to the (personified) rationality of the illness. To the tune of: "Come on, leave. Elsewhere is so much more pleasant than here." We employ powers of persuasion instead of giving orders in this case.

Persuasion spells present a good alternative for those of you who are having a hard time with spells phrased as commands for your personal taste.

> *Good evening, Old Woman,*
> *I am bringing you the warm and the cold.*

…meaning warm and cold fevers (chills or shivers). Find a tree for this spell. This can be an oak tree, elder tree, apple tree, nut tree, spruce, or willow tree.

A similar spell utilizes a crossroads instead of a tree as a magical space. To perform this kind of magic, go to a crossroads and say:

> *Good day, crossroads!*
> *I am bringing you my warmth and my cold.*
> *I am leaving the cold with you;*
> *I am keeping my warmth.*[20]

Afterward, walk home in silence without turning back.

It's interesting how we again reference ancient magical ideas: the crossroads is addressed like a person. We know from ancient times and other cultures that some deities liked to linger at crossroads, especially gods of fate that can open or close paths in life.

---

20. Frischbier, 53

Dislocations, Sprains, Joint Problems, etc.

St. Peter sat on a stone
And he had a bad leg.
Flesh and flesh, blood and blood,
In three days it will be good.

This spell is very reminiscent of the Second Merseburg Charm, except it uses St. Peter instead of Wodan, who healed the blood, limb, and joint dislocations in that particular magic spell with the following words:

Bone to bone; blood to blood;
Limb to limb—like they were glued.

These similarities are no coincidence. This is where an age-old form of the magic spell mixes with the more modern view of Christianity (St. Peter).

Spells against dislocations can easily be used for joint problems and even for rheumatism. The limb in this spell stands for all extremities, so the spell will work well on an arm or anywhere else it is needed.

It is not uncommon for healing spells to be applied to ailments for which they were never intended. Ancient healers who used prayers knew a spell or two, yet people came to them with other ailments in their times of need. The known spells were applied to these ailments or new ones were thought up. What else can one do in times of need?

No relatively open exchange existed for topics like these. There was always the fear of being accused of practicing witchcraft. It has been suggested that the two World Wars were primarily responsible for the distribution of spells in recent history. Healers who entered the army often recognized each other when one of them stopped a bleeding or lessened pain, more or less in secret, for their comrades. They would then trade healing knowledge. This also happened often among refugees and displaced people during those wars.

Dizziness

I talk off your dizziness.
You will wind
From skin and hair,
From flesh and blood,
From marrow and limb,
You shall not be dizzy
Even as little as the stone.[21]

During this sympathetic cure a stone with healing powers is held above the forehead and then returned to its proper place at the end.

Dizziness, dizziness, dizziness, you torture me,
Dizziness, dizziness, dizziness, I hunt you,
Dizziness, dizziness, dizziness, you shall disappear.[22]

The magic moment in this spell is the triple address; the rest is clearly a call to battle.

Flesh and blood
Skin and limb
Stand like stone.

Spells against dizziness were not exclusively used for healing treatments, but would also be spoken to ensure a good head for heights when traveling in the mountains or higher altitudes.

---

21. Atkinson-Scarter, 91
22. Hampp, 78

Eczema

The eczema category includes psoriasis, neurodermatitis, and all other skin conditions that result in scales. Dandruff can also be considered one of them.

If a skin problem appears in the form of redness or heat, use a spell against burns. As soon as scales form on the skin, however, use a spell against eczema, even if the skin shows redness. Traditional healing medicine suggests salt water as an additional compress to heal eczema. Today many people resort to seawater applications or to creating their own "sea" water—by mixing sea salt and water.

> *Eczema, eczema, go away!*
> *My hands chase you.*
> *They chase you day and night,*
> *So, eczema, eczema, eczema,*
> *Go away from me!*[23]

This spell delivers a clear statement and chases off the eczema. The mental image in this spell is clear. It is easy to imagine two hands chasing after the eczema to drive it away.

> *Eczema, step down from the backside,*
> *From the backside to the heel,*
> *From the heel to the ground.*[24]

This spell serves as a kind of lightning rod spell. The eczema is sent down the body and finally grounded in the Earth, which takes it on and neutralizes it. This spell can be easily changed to work for other illnesses.

Two other relatively well-known spells work with the motif of no return:

---

23. Hampp, 79
24. Hampp, 80

The moon and eczema
Walk across the water;
The moon returns home,
Eczema stays away.

Fly ash and eczema
Flew across the sea;
Fly ash returns home,
Eczema is never seen again.

Fly ash—in other variations of this spell also defined as flake ash or potash—is ash that is fine enough to be airborne. In the old days it was used directly and was symbolically blown away or applied to the affected area. Some sources[25] also list fly ash as ash from beech wood.

It was easy to work this way back when people had wood-burning ovens in their homes. Today it is often easier to take dried herbs such as rosemary, stinging nettle, or ragweed, burn them on a fireproof surface, then use the resultant ash and repeat this either three or nine times:

Evil eczema, go back home.

Spells can be just that simple! This is a clear statement without any embellishment used to banish eczema.

The Evil Eye, Jinxing

(today: Mobbing, Workplace Bullying)

In the old days, people often assumed that envy, sinister thinking, and sometimes even excessive admiration could cause an illness. These ailments were often treated with spells.

We still know the feeling when an illness first comes on: something's got a hold of me. Envy has a powerful energy. It does not necessarily have to have evil intention, even if the expression evil eye sounds like

---

25. Schmidt, 89

it. It often happens unknowingly and without intent. In general, we shouldn't expect an attack behind everything, so just discreetly and quietly resolve the problem without any drama or accusations.

> *Friend, if you are cursed in your leg,*
> *And in your lungs,*
> *And in your liver,*
> *If an evil woman has done it to you,*
> *Or if a young girl has done it to you,*
> *Or if an evil man has done it to you,*
> *Or if a young boy has done it to you,*
> *So bring it home to them*
> *In their lung and their liver,*
> *Let it stick there forever.*

Most spells against the evil eye show this typical list of questions, in which all potential candidates that could have caused it are being considered. Since the source of the energy can only be directly traced back in the rarest of cases, it was a safety measure to ensure that no possible instigator was left out of consideration.

This spell can be used today to bring clarity to cases of defamation, bullying, etc. The sorrow that results from such problems almost always has a physical effect, such as sleep troubles or stomach aches. When we look at it from this perspective, we can understand what it means when we say that the charm of certain people can do bodily damage. If you consider the last two lines of the spell too extreme, you may leave it off and end the spell with "so bring it home to them." It is simply the language from another time.

> *Who cursed you?*
> *Their own kidneys will feel it.*
> *Who cursed you, man or woman?*
> *They will feel it themselves.*

Who has cursed you, lass or lad?
They will feel sick themselves.

This spell is a classic: the bad intentions will be returned to sender. Let them cope with their own bitterness instead of afflicting their acquaintances! Less personal banishments also existed that were not phrased quite so harshly. For instance:

Evil eye, evil eye,
Go to the lonely mountain,
Where the birds do not sing,
Where no man can go.[26]

The culprit is not named directly with this banishment, but the evil eye itself is banished without involving the sender. The previous spell was in the form of mirrored intent (meaning that negativity is returned to the sender). Here, the evil eye is personified and sent away without targeting a specific person.

Two evil eyes cursed you;
Two good eyes call you back.

This fairly well-known spell comes right to the point and sets things straight. The old folk beliefs contained not only the evil eye, but a good eye as well. It had healing properties and could return things to balance.

Female Troubles

In the old days people believed that the uterus had a life of its own. It was viewed as an animal (usually a toad) that was believed to have the ability to wander around inside the body, which caused considerable discomfort.

---

26. Hampp, 92

Today we are aware that this is not true and view these analogies in a different light. In order to feel healthy, the magical cauldron of a woman's belly has to be in good shape! These old spells can also be successfully applied to menstrual pain and PMS.

Once again, we shouldn't fall victim to mindless, ideological thinking here. It is often believed, especially in spiritual circles, that menstrual pain indicates that a woman is not on the best terms with her femininity. Let's not be ridiculous. Menstruation is the shedding of the uterine lining in the body, and the body naturally feels this when it happens. Of course, we can and should lessen the pain this causes, but to add feelings of guilt to the process is absolutely … questionable, to put it mildly. In the old days women were considered unclean when they had their period. Today we assume they are not sufficiently enlightened when they are in pain. It's enough to drive anyone mad.

> *Old woman—old cat*
> *Drink a little glass of schnapps!*
> *Womb, stop toying with me like a cat.*[27]

This spell is obviously a drinking spell that was aimed at soothing the uterus with a little drink of schnapps. It will also work with tea or another helpful remedy instead of the alcohol.

Many women prefer to suffer in silence during their period instead of taking "evil" pharmaceutical medications. To each her own, but why play the martyr when you could be having a nice day?

Naturally, medications should be used responsibly and sparingly. Ask your doctor or pharmacist about best practices. When you see no other way, this is by no means an option that would turn you into an unspiritual person.

The spells were not always as peaceful as the previous one. Sometimes they took a different tone:

---

27. Hampp, 60

Uterus, rest now!
If you move,
I'll kill you.

We can clearly imagine the uterus as an animal within the body in this spell. It is supposed to keep to a certain area. This is accomplished through an obvious threat. Any woman who has ever suffered from strong menstruation pains can understand this drastic language. The following spell is even clearer:

Mother I dam you.
Mother I clamp you.
Mother go to your place
Where the Lord has destined you.[28]

The traveling uterus is supposed to return to her designated place to restore inner order.

Woe-mother, bear-mother,
You want to lick blood,
To repel the heart,
To strain the limbs,
To stretch the skin,
You mustn't do it;
You must rest.

This blessing travels through the entire body; the restless uterus is being soothed and put into its place. This is not done with threats, but in a soothing manner. This is a useful spell even from today's perspective. After all, menstruation can put an unpleasant strain on many parts

---

28. Hampp, 59. Note: in this spell, "mother" is short for "bear-mother" (Gebärmutter), the German word for womb or uterus. (The "bear" in the word refers to bearing children, not the animal.)

of the body when we consider side effects such as headaches, nausea, cramps, diarrhea, and a funky feeling in general.

Growths

Growth, you paw of a dog,
You grew big as an apple,
From apple to nut,
From nut to bean,
From bean to pea,
From pea to poppy seed,
From poppy seed to nothing.
So the growth shall also vanish,
As does
Foam on the sea,
Dew on the grass,
Wax on the fire.[29]

This spell has a special form that relies on invoking a step-by-step reduction, which eventually leads to the elimination of the problem. This form can be very inspiring if you are thinking about inventing your own spells.

Our ancestors' spells were never complicated. They are always phrased in clear language that is hard to misunderstand. There is no beating around the bush, like "Maybe I would like to experience a little healing, but only if I remain in balance with my karmic duties and responsibilities and do not go against my guru's master plan." Healing spells have to make a clear statement if they are to be effective. Every restriction and "but," "maybe," or "if," no matter how small, disrupts, and scatters the power.

As I mentioned above, faith includes the belief that we have a right to be healed. Those who doubt this and who are of the opinion that they have forfeited the right to healing based on personal badness, guilt,

---

29. Hampp, 37

karma, sin, or similar things, must deal with this mental construction zone before they can work with healing spells. Spells can only unfold their full effect when they are spoken fully, with trust and confidence.

Gout, Rheumatism, and Similar Pain

Good evening, Spruce,
Take away my gout.
Rheumatism and rupture
Shall yield from my body.[30]

This spell originated in Brandenburg; its motif, however, can be found in all regions, in which illnesses are addressed: folks go to a so-called "storing" tree with their illness and turn over the illness to the tree.

Elders also fall into the storing tree category:

Elder shrub, I shake you,
Elder shrub, I quake you,
I, N.N., quake and shake to you
My seventy-seven forms of gout.

Spells that incorporate trees as healing entities are relatively well known and easy to find. This suggests a significant prevalence among the population. It appears that they were not only used by healers, but were considered public property and as such used to help people when needed.

Ultimately, all spells in which an illness is chased off into the woods are tied to the faith that considers trees to have helping powers:

Gout, I command you
Out of the head and out of the throat,
Out of the flesh and out of the limb,

---

30. Hampp, 87

Out of the blood and out of the marrow,
Into a desolate and wild wood,
Where neither sun nor moon shine anymore.[31]

This spell can be used for more than gout. The first word "gout" can be exchanged for any illness, since the spell works its way through the entire body. It is not tailored to a specific ailment.

Headaches

Headache, go away,
Fling yourself onto a dead body
And leave the living alone.

This spell involves those who have passed away, which may seem to lack reverence for the dead at first glance. These spells are not meant to disturb the deceased or overwhelm them with illnesses, however, but to state a simple analogy: as the dead fade away, so the illness shall fade. "It doesn't hurt the dead. They're already dead," a healer once remarked.

In Wehlau (Saxony Anhalt) headaches were referred to as "little people." They were believed to be a kind of sickness spirit akin to goblins or worms. Ash was supposed to be good medicine against them, especially if it was collected during the Twelve Nights (the magical nights between Christmas and Epiphany). The following spell also brought relief:

You little people,
You dear people,
All of you!
Go out of the head,
Go out of body and limb,
Go to the water, where you will find a broad stone,
There you will find food and drink.[32]

---

31. Hampp, 92
32. Frischbier, 75

This spell was performed at the water. Afterward one would make three banishing crosses in the water with a knife, and walk away. A modern variation is to fill a sink with water and let the water drain out of the sink after drawing the three crosses. This works wonderfully well.

The little people were elsewhere known as "white" or "cold" people because they turned the affected person white, meaning pale and cold as they made them sick and weak. This banishing formula is suitable for all circumstances in which people are unwell in general and may look a little pale around the gills. Of course, it also reminds us that white is traditionally the color of spirits, and "dear people" represent the spirit of an illness. At the very least they are spirits occupying the wrong place and need to be banished. We often find shamanic views on illnesses which survived in these spells to the current day.

An old Romany spell against headaches goes like this:

> *Pain, oh pain in my head!*
> *The father of all evil*
> *Will find you, cursed pain.*
> *Travel on, be smart;*
> *You have tortured me enough!*
> *There is neither seat nor bed for you here,*
> *I want to chase you from my head!*
> *Where you once were nursed*
> *Travel back there, you evil thing!*
> *Whoever steps in my shadow*
> *Possess his head instead.*[33]

The line "where you once were nursed" represents a clear order: Go home to Mommy.

This spell makes use of yet another healing technique: transference. This is most likely a later addition, and actually weakens the spell. The

---

33. Von Wlislocki: *Folk Beliefs and Religious Customs of the Gypsies*, 61

headache is now unsure whether it is supposed to go home to Mommy or torture another through magical transference (via the shadow).

While the technique of transference is not exactly the way of the proper English gentleman, it was often practiced in the olden days. An illness was often transferred via a coin, for instance, because unattended money is quickly picked up.

It is a handy spell to have, although we can omit the last two lines. They do not agree with the modern understanding of magic and they make the spell somewhat ambiguous. This isn't helpful in healing practices.

Muscle Tension, Muscle Hardening, Knots

Muscle knot from the head,
The best horse to the manger!
If it won't help,
It won't harm either. [34]

Afterward one would blow three times across the tense body part, like a shoulder (the shoulders are indicated with "from the head" in this spell).

Another spell from regions of Northern Germany:

A stag without lung,
A stork without tongue,
A turtle dove without gall,
Muscle knots, fall (off).

These two spells leave many mysteries and as modern thinking people we tend to want to analyze what could be behind it. From my own experience, do yourself a favor and accept what might work for you, but don't analyze it to death. The old spells have a completely different force field, and it fades away when we try to dissect it with our minds.

I found a very similar spell against fever with a slight change:

---

34. Schmidt, 87, the following spell: 88

Frogs without lung,

Storks without tongue,

Fish without gall,

Take my seventy-seven fevers all! [35]

The first variation finds its origin on the island of Rügen, the second originated in Werder near Berlin. As you can see they were used for entirely different ailments. The second spell in particular can be applied to any other illness without a problem.

Nightmares

God protect me from the nightmare!

With all your might.

Wade through all the waters,

Leaf through all the trees,

Cross all boundaries,

Cut through the grease,

Count all the little stars in the sky,

Count all the little grains of sand in the seas,

Count all planks and fences,

Count all shingles on the roof.

In the meantime, the dear day will come around;

The nightmare can't squeeze me.[36]

This spell is typical for a preoccupation formula, in which one keeps the evil spirit that causes the nightmare busy, so it will not disturb you. (The German word for nightmare, *Alptraum,* is derived from the word *alp,* a spirit being that would press or squeeze a person at night. Also known as a pressure ghost or incubus.)

Any kind of fringe on clothing serves as similar protection to preoccupation spells because ghosts have to count all of them, which affords

---

35. Frischbier, 54

36. Hampp, 101

the person peace and quiet for a little while. In the African American magic tradition people used to glue newspapers to the walls because spirits have to read all of it before they can do anything else. Similar ideas exist in countless cultures. Our ancestors were familiar with them as well.

Rasђ

The term rash covers a variety of skin conditions. The following spell covers all bases:

> *I will bless off the bothersome rash of the so baptized N.N, three times nine pimples, three times nine pustules, and three times nine exanthems. The mother of God walked along a green bridge and found three herbs. She picked one with her right hand; she wrapped the second around her right foot, and lost the third. No one knows where it went. Let these exanthems of the so baptized N.N. disappear in the same way, without known destination. Not through mine, mine, mine, but through the help of Lord Jesus and all the Saints.*[37]

Stressing the act of baptism in this spell no doubt serves to activate the healing powers in these terms: "Mary and Jesus take notice … you are obligated to help this person." Of course, you can leave out the word baptism and add your own spiritual helpers to the spell. All of these spells were invented at one time or another and we have the same right to do so as our ancestors.

We often have a funny relationship with things we invent because we feel that it does not hold the validity in some way—it's just not real.

That is such nonsense. (Other cultures are a lot more relaxed and invent more as a result.) The ability to invent something is a gift and we would be misguided not to use it. Not a single healing blessing would have been created if no one had thought of it at some point. Our heads do not exist just for haircuts.

---

37. Frischbier, 35

The Rose

As I mentioned earlier, "the rose" (a broad category of rashes or erysipelas) is a subcategory of a burn. However, several spells exist that are specifically tailored to this ailment.

> *The rose and the willow*
> *Had a quarrel;*
> *The willow won,*
> *The rose disappeared.*

The willow as a healing tree, in which people often symbolically hung illnesses, stands as victor over the rose. This spell was also passed down for eczema. In this case simply use the word eczema instead of rose for this spell.

> *Three virgins wandered the land.*
> *One picks leaves,*
> *The other picks grass,*
> *The third breaks the rose.*

Another variation of this spell goes like this:

> *Three virgins wandered along green paths.*
> *One picks flowers,*
> *Another one picks lilies,*
> *The third drives the rose away.*

These poetic spells conjure up a clear mental image. We also run into our three holy women again.

> *Rose, do not prick,*
> *Rose, do not break,*
> *Rose, do not stay,*
> *Rose, wither away.*

This spell is relatively well known and belongs to the most frequently used spells against the rose.

A rock stands in the red sea.
On it stands a made-up bed covered in cotton linens,
There you, rosy perforated ulcer
Have a space to sleep.
Sleep and rest until judgment day.[38]

We have encountered this persuasive type of spell before, in which we offer the illness another, more beautiful place to be, as opposed to giving it an eviction order. Here we offer the rose a "bed covered in cotton linens" as a comfortable living space. The spell still retains a little bit of an order in its tone. The rose is supposed to sleep there and rest (so, by no means even think about wandering around!). We are dealing with a mixed form here, using gentle force.

The "red sea" can supposedly be interpreted as a psychological interpretation of blood or a symbol for new strength. However, I think it serves as a biblical reference to Moses, who parted the Red Sea. It could also be much simpler than that: Because the Red Sea was far away, the illness is also banished to a faraway place. We will likely never know what was meant exactly, because we would have to be able to ask the inventor of the spell directly.

The rose and the dragon
Wandered across the creek.
The rose vanished,
The dragon drowned.[39]

A healer from Berlin was the source for this spell. Like many folk healers, she traced the origin of the rose back to a shock or a psychologically

---

38. Hampp, 98
39. Bühring, 96

stressful situation—hence the dragon. It symbolizes the moment of fright, which is banished as the root of all evil to ensure the rose does not return.

Spells against the rose are also effective against herpes, especially if it persists over a long period of time or keeps reappearing in short periods. Those who suffer from cold sores on or around the mouth know that they often appear during stressful times or can be sparked by a moment of fright (such as a disgusting or seemingly fearsome sight). This is the same cause that folk healers also assume for a break-out of the rose. If this is the case for you, you can use the spells exactly as they are. No need to substitute the word herpes for rose.

We can also use these spells for other dermatological illnesses when we do not have anything else handy. Many traditional suggestions hold true against the rose. Do not let it come in contact with water, but apply warm compresses with dry chamomile buds. These can be wrapped in a thin cotton cloth (like a cotton diaper), warmed in the oven or on a radiator and then gently applied.

Soothing Pain

The wound happened,
Now and in the hour,
May it not bleed,
Not hurt,
Not fester,
Not ulcerate,
Until the mother of God gives birth to a second son.

In short, the last line "until the mother of God gives birth to a second son" means: never. It is a popular ending for blessings that are meant to banish a condition once and for all.

In many blessings we find the word "not," a negative statement. Many find this strange today, since the latest teachings in spiritual circles preach that you must not say "not." The reason for this is supposedly the brain cannot process "not," or just skips over it, which either leaves the undesired condition to remain or possibly even strengthens it. Our ancestors obviously saw this differently and did pretty well with it.

We should be careful not to exaggerate principles like this, but to consider things realistically. We all know the sobering effect of the sentence "You can NOT do that." I have yet to meet someone who considers this sentence (as the "not-theory" would suggest) as a strengthening statement. The opposite is true: it tends to drag people down and is disheartening. Many fight against statements like this their entire life. This effectively shows how powerful negative comments can be. The little word "not" has a powerful effect. It draws boundaries for good and for ill.

I come to you, flood of water,
I offer you my fury against the hurt.
Take it into the deep sand,
Lead it into a foreign land.

This spell would clearly work best if spoken by a flowing body of water, thereby incorporating the water's energy.

If such a body of water is not present or the person whom you are trying to support cannot go to one, you can easily speak the spell with a mental image of a flowing body of water that carries the pain away. You can also use a bowl of water and let it run down the drain at the end. A postcard of a river or a waterfall can also be helpful if the person can hardly move or is bedridden. A little creativity is sometimes necessary.

Traditional healers are generally very careful when it comes to soothing pain. They often go to work only after a doctor has examined things and has determined a diagnosis (because it is critical to know the exact kind of pain). It would not be very helpful, for instance, if one tried to soothe the pain of appendicitis, since its cause would not be eliminated this way.

Stress and Similar Conditions

Our ancestors certainly experienced some stress, but their worries primarily centered around physical health and the dangers that threatened life and limb. Nevertheless, spells against fright, terror, and similar conditions exist, like the following spell. These can be used for heightened stress and mental ailments.

Take off, fright!
The mother's breath
And the father's strength chase you
Into a grey horse,
Into the straw of rye
Into a moldering tree trunk.[40]

This spell originated in Bosnia; as is the case with many traditions in folk magic, fright—meaning a specific moment of stress or a traumatizing situation—is seen as the source of the resulting illness.

Our German folk magic also assumes fright, as well as the evil eye, as a catalyst for illness. This is a worldwide motif that also appears in the South American healing tradition, for example. The belief that we should spit after a frightful moment to guard against illness persists even today.

Toothaches

Toothaches take up a large part of the old healing traditions and we count ourselves lucky to be able to have access to modern dental practices.

One of the old stories from the Alps tells of a man who lies screaming and moaning on the ground because he broke his leg. He encounters a dwarf, who asks him why he is screaming so loud and the man points to his leg. The dwarf answers unconcerned: "Oh, is that it? The way you were screaming, I thought you had a toothache."

---

40. Hampp, 95

Even if no one enjoys a trip to the dentist, this story very clearly demonstrates how things looked in the past. People considered the pain of broken bones harmless in comparison to a toothache.

I am mentioning the following spells merely for historical reasons. We all know that we should immediately see a doctor when we have a toothache—and even better, before one develops.

> *Welcome bright light*
> *For the teeth and for the gout.*
> *Take all my little worms*
> *That eat at my limbs.*[41]

Most of the spells that have been found about toothaches welcome the light, meaning the new day. We can therefore assume that these spells were spoken at sunrise.

> *Greetings, new light*
> *With your two points!*
> *My teeth should not twinge*
> *Until you have three points.*[42]

This spell may have been spoken at the time of the new crescent moon, again welcoming new light. A crescent moon has two points, so the final line— "until you have three points"—means "never," just as we saw in the spell for soothing pain that said, "until the mother of God gives birth to a second son."

Universal Banishing and Prevention

> *Holy Mother Mary moves through the land,*
> *With nine (name the disease) in her hand.*
> *If she does not have nine, she has eight,*

---

41. Schmidt, 105

42. Frischbier, 100

If she does not have eight, she has seven,
If she does not have seven, she has six,
If she does not have six, she has five,
If she does not have five, she has four,
If she does not have four, she has three,
If she does not have three, she has two,
If she does not have two, she has one,
If she does not have one, she has none.[43]

This magic spell was originally spoken to prevent illnesses of the eye; however, it can be applied to any other ailment. Its form is reminiscent of classical magic spells, in which one letter is sequentially omitted for the purpose of banishing, as well known from the "Abracadabra" formula, the meaning of which is still wrapped in secrecy:

Abracadabra
Abracadabr
Abracadab
Abracada
Abracad
Abraca
Abrac
Abra
Abr
Ab
A

In this case the illness is reduced until it has disappeared. This spell is very powerful and easy to remember. One should always keep it in mind because you never know when it will come in handy.

The following spell originates from the folk beliefs of the Hungarian Roma and speaks to the new crescent moon, meaning the phase in which

---

43. See: Fehrle, 60

you can see the first fine sliver of a crescent (the new light). Healers spoke to the crescent moon to prevent or relieve illnesses for one phase of the moon (the spell lasts this long and has to be repeated afterward):

New moon, new king!
Give me graciously
Good weeks,
In good weeks
Good days,
In good days
Good hours,
In good hours
Good fortune,
And keep me well
And healthy! [44]

We have seen that reduction in spells is meant to banish illnesses; here the method of reduction is used to drill down to the shortest span of time, so as to not leave anything out. This spell serves well when made into a monthly habit, spoken on the second or third day after the astronomical new moon (when the moon is in complete darkness).

The crescent moon (when the new light is visible) was also used to increase money. This is why it is good to have a few coins in your pocket at this time. When you see the new moon for the first time, rattle the coins in your pocket with a wish for more. It may not bring an instant lotto win, but it almost always leads to unexpected gains during the lunar month.

Warts

Let that which I here talk off
Pass;
Let that with which I talk it off
Last. [45]

---

44. Von Wlislocki: *Magic Formulas and Incantations …*, 24
45. Bühring, 97

Another spell goes like this:

> *What I see passes,*
> *What I strike yields.*

This form of treatment is fairly common: tie as many knots in a string as there are warts and bury it, so it decomposes. Be mindful to use a string made of natural fibers, otherwise it cannot decompose.

Rubbing bacon on the warts and burying it afterward is also a proven method. Occasionally it says to bury the bacon in a graveyard; this again follows the idea of the illness vanishing just as corpses rot away. This is not necessary and certainly not for everyone, but it can't hurt.

The old household remedies against warts are still popular today. An old friend from school told me to sprinkle urine on a wart when the moon is full to make it disappear. This is not an absurd idea when we consider that many crèmes contain urea as an ingredient. It works well, has no side effects, doesn't hurt, and it's free. And you don't have to tell anyone about it, after all.

Worms

In traditional healing medicine worms are by no means considered simply as the actual parasites within the human body that they are, but are also viewed as sickness spirits as I have already explained. Today we would describe them as energy thieves or bad vibes.

> *Three kings plow a field.*
> *What do they plow up?*
> *They plow up three little worms;*
> *The first one was white,*
> *The second one was yellow,*
> *The third one was red,*
> *I squeeze them with my five fingers to death.*[46]

---

46. Hampp, 67

Some spells (even when they refer to other illnesses) either work through the entire color palette or they target very specific colors that are connected to the illness. The thought behind this was to be careful not to forget any form of the illness to avoid giving it a loophole that would allow it to stay.

> *Worm and she-worm,*
> *I forbid you to touch the human.*
> *His flesh and his blood,*
> *His marrow and his limbs,*
> *You shall die and never come alive again.*[47]

The fun ends when dealing with worms. The spells make this very clear. The interesting part about this spell is that it addresses the male and female worm as a pair. That makes sense; both sexes are necessary for procreation. This blessing targets not only the destruction of the worms, but also indirectly addresses their multiplication.

---

47. Hampp, 69

Powerful Plants

We have the option of working with hundreds of thousands of plants to help our healing processes. I had to make some choices for this chapter and bumped into my first dilemma: what exactly is a *native* plant? Plants themselves cannot wander, but seem to enjoy using humans to do so. The medicine of monastic gardens exemplified many Mediterranean plants, which were considered exotic back then. Today they are a staple known to any herbal witch. As a result, I am sticking to plants that are both commonly used today and have also been established for centuries in my part of Europe.

It was important to me that many of the plants be well known; they are easy to find, and you can plant or forage them yourself. What use are fancy plants if barely anyone has the opportunity to enjoy working with them in practice? My preference in my selection for this book was to provide a solid "best of" versus a show of rarities.

Many books talk about compounds or active constituents when it comes to healing work with plants. They are right to do so, since this is an important part of their healing powers. However, plants do not only possess a body that contains specific compounds. They also have a soul, a spirit that can be addressed. This goes hand in hand with their physical properties.

We can still feel this knowledge in the old lore. People used to wear plants as holy amulets, which targets the spirit of the plant, since this was neither an internal application (like tea) nor a topical application (like a salve). It was meant to bring harmony to the entire energy field of the sick person. In today's terminology, we'd say that the plant's energy is absorbed into the aura of the patient.

People smoked plants, and they were also popular as infusions to baths, especially during the traditional spring spa times that were supervised by a bath woman or man. These baths were meant to drive winter and the resulting "bad juices" from the body in order to renew the body as nature renews itself in the spring.

Today we commonly believe Plant A has active constituents 1, 2, and 3, and as a result it works against ailments a, b, and c. This is not how spiritual medicine works because it relies on the personal connection to a plant. People may feel a connection to some plants, but not to others. Figuratively speaking, some plants have a similar temperature to us (instead of temperature we can also say: vibration, color, aura—depending on which channel of perception you happen to personally feel it). If one has become unbalanced due to stress or illness, the plant serves as a reminder to the body how it feels when it is in harmony with itself.

In the following descriptions of plants, I made sure to include the energetic and magical powers of plants, too. I see this as a suggestion to delve deeper into the subject. One's relationship with healing plants should be based on love. This does not mean disregarding all the knowledge about their biochemical healing properties, just that they are simply not everything. When I describe the spiritual effects of the plant, it should only be viewed as an inspiration: it is my point of view. Yours may be entirely different. I don't want to tell anyone how they should feel about a plant. This text should be viewed as an introduction that you can expand for yourself.

The body emits clear signals about what it wants. All we have to do is pay close attention to it. If people would forego vitamin supplements and listen to their appetites instead, their body would receive exactly what it needs. A healthy appetite is something entirely instinctual; we are rarely brave enough to listen to our instincts or animalistic nature as the old healers called it. This is similar when it comes to healing plants, which is why we should ask ourselves during their selection: "Which plant do I crave?" This also applies to healing baths or body oils.

You can always reference guidebooks and spreadsheets afterward, but initially you should go with your intuition.

We cannot strictly organize plants by assigning them to specific problems. It is only when we listen to our gut feelings that we truly free our intuition—or our access to it, since it is technically always there and knows what is good for us. In other words, you will need to learn to sense like an animal again, to know which leaf is good for you and which one is not. This is not something the head can do alone. Intuition has a lot to do with it, as well as experience.

This does not fall from the sky. It wants to be (re)learned. Without experience we simply cannot compare. No matter how long you try to describe how a plant smells, tastes, or acts, if you have not experienced it yourself you cannot understand or relate to it.

When it comes to the subject of healing we are bombarded by so many alleged truths, studies, and statistics that we have a hard time with the most natural approach. In the meantime, simply go within and *feel* instead of listening to the hyped-up chatter of the health market in order to find the truth within yourself. This requires a change in our way of thinking: do not simply feed the head with data, but let your instincts speak: our natural sense for that which is good for us and that which is not.

Even supposedly "good" things may not be good for us all the time. Perhaps you have experienced this yourself? When you work with a plant long enough—drinking its tea, for example—you will feel it eventually: "I don't really enjoy this anymore. It feels stale." Recognizing when your body tries to tell you something and taking it seriously is an important task.

We often treat our bodies like strangers or even worse—like someone who has no clue, something that is simply stupid matter, but luckily ruled by an intelligent, radiant spirit. But naturally, our body speaks to us physically. Not a single case of burnout would exist if it were customary to listen to what our bodies tells us. We will get the bill for our ignorance and delusions of grandeur (what else can we call the notion that we have limitless energy?) eventually.

I would like to address a common misunderstanding in regard to herbal studies: Some people still believe that "a lot helps a lot" or believe that they should or must take a greater amount of herbs because herbs are a) not as strong or b) made up of pure nature and therefore harmless. A little more respect, please! Herbs have a very real effect and can therefore—like anything that works—have side effects as well. Especially pregnant women, diabetics, and all those that are physically in an unusual situation should consult a physician or healer with the appropriate expertise to educate themselves about which herbs to use.

If you are planning on consulting a doctor, first find out how much they know about healing plants. Then you won't have the experience that an acquaintance of mine had when he asked his doctor if he could use valerian instead of a sleeping pill for relaxation. The answer he received was, "Valerian does not work. It only has an effect on women and cats." Your pharmacist may be the better contact person, also, when it comes to the effects and interactions of plants and medications.

I personally work with herbs as givers of impulses. That means that I do not consider them a remedy in the sense of "this substance will bring the body back to health," but rather "they give the body the impulse to return itself back to health." Often we end up somewhere in the middle and the plant heals specifically through its acting compounds that set the body back on its path by mobilizing it to heal itself.

In the following section I will introduce important healing plants and a few of their possible areas of application. I am deliberately adding a few normal kitchen recipes in which magical plants play a leading role. Our ancestors did not consider cooking and medicine to be separate areas. Consider the books written by Hildegard von Bingen. I purposely chose to provide comfort food rather than "health food" recipes (whatever is currently touted as being "healthy") because indulgence in moderation simply does the body good, and unites body and soul. Even Goethe said: "No pleasure is temporary, because the impression it leaves is permanent."

At the end of this chapter I will then provide the most common methods on how to prepare these plants in detail.

One more important tip: Plants that are labeled with the following icon should not be consumed during pregnancy: ⊘

Angelica ⊘
(Angelica archangelica)

Angelica, often called "Angel Root" in German (and formerly in English as well), is a healing plant full of light, which becomes apparent because it renders its user sensitive to light, similar to St. John's wort. You should therefore avoid sunbathing and take care to use good sun protection after consumption.

Angelica is mostly found in herbal liqueurs or in candied form in sweets.

Angel Root has become a bit of a forgotten thing in our area. It is more often used as a fumigant than a healing plant. It is still held in high honors elsewhere, however.

During my research for this book I ended up in Iceland, where angelica is primarily consumed as a tea and in capsules, juices, and even in skin care products. It is supposed to prevent memory loss, bring harmony to the heart and circulation, soothe infections, fight colds and bronchitis, reduce fungus and bacteria, soothe the stomach, prevent motion sickness, revive the skin, soothe eczema and psoriasis, and curtail headaches, rheumatism, and illnesses of the joints. After reading all of these recommendations, I had to ask myself what illness could not be cured with angelica? Even severe illnesses were on the list. The people of Iceland believe the things that carried our Viking ancestors through bitterly cold winters can still awaken our elementary powers today.

The plant grows on every corner in Iceland, which is another valuable hint; be consciously interested in which plants grow close to you (even if you live in the city) and what their healing properties may be. We can usually say a lot about a place and its energy by the plants that are found there.

Angelica is recommended for colds in our area as well, especially against stubborn coughs. It acts as an expectorant and simultaneously strengthens the immune system, therefore fighting the deeper cause of the infection. Angelica stems used to be tied around the chest in the form of a cross—the so-called chest cross—to ban colds.

Angelica is also a proven stomach soother. It should be carefully dosed since it packs a lot of power. Drink the tea one sip at a time and see how it feels internally. Do not listen blindly to recommendations; a lot of it is a matter of individual tolerance (black tea and coffee does not agree with everyone either, for example).

Angelica is a valuable root against bewitched illnesses, especially as an antidote against magically-induced impotence. This problem occurs less frequently today, although as witches we still receive spell requests from women that want their partner to run in top form for them alone, not other ladies. Some wishes simply prove to be timeless, since the topic is not completely off the table even in the twenty-first century.

On an emotional level angelica is an extremely powerful plant. Work with it whenever you can't see the light at the end of the tunnel, either in tea form or in herbal sachets carried on the body. In awkward, difficult situations in which you are faced with a "dark" force, regardless of whether it's a boss or a mother-in-law, angelica offers the best of services. It is a powerful plant that embodies both light and strength.

Protection Pouch

This protection pouch has a spiritual effect and can be used in any difficult situation (including health-related ones), as a companion on the way to the doctor's office or the hospital for example.

You will need:

Black fabric (nothing synthetic)

Red string

Angelica root

St. John's wort

Oak (bark, leaves—whatever you can find)

A piece of coral or some other red stone

Lay out the ingredients on the black cloth cut in the form of a circle. If black makes you uncomfortable you can choose another color (violet or dark red, for example). I recommend black because it is a classic color of protection.

Angelica root and St. John's wort provide protection, light, and power. The oak adds steadfastness in the storms of life. The red stone and coral strengthen vitality and the will to persevere. Before you tie it up, look at everything quietly. You can meditate with it or speak a prayer or your goals above it. Words are ingredients as well.

Afterward, tie up the pouch with the red string and make three knots. Carry it with you or have it close by when you can't wear it on you.

Anise

(Pimpinella anisum)

Anise is primarily known as a remedy for stomach pains, whether it is a feeling of being full or nauseous in adults or stomach twinges with the little ones. It has a balancing effect on the entire gastrointestinal tract; it removes toxins from the body and has a relaxing effect. It can soothe a baby's digestion troubles through the mother's milk. The nursing mother simply needs to drink the tea. Anise is often recommended to new mothers and pregnant women as a remedy that brings harmony to the body.

Anise also helps to drain discharge during colds, which restores breathing. It is a first-rate tonic that allows new strength to grow and has a lovely aroma compared to many bitter or tart herbal plants. Anise provides inner light in dark times and is considered a plant that promotes a bright outlook. It further protects against the evil eye and nightmares, as do almost all aromatic plants. Anise is also an aphrodisiac.

Baked goods with anise were once used as a popular offering during spring and fall in Northern Germany, meaning at the beginning and end of the agricultural work. Women coaxed men out of their shells with anise-flavored drinks. All things considered, anise is a plant that reaffirms the joy of life. It harmonizes, relaxes, and brings light. As such it should be a staple in any witch's herbal pharmacy.

The plant spirit of anise is cheerful, light, exhilarating, sweet, lovely, and medicinal. This power is often underappreciated, but as they say, those who do not savor will become unsavory. What good is it to work sixty hours a week and drive an expensive car when all you can do is come home and fall into bed exhausted without time to appreciate your hard-earned money? Important key concepts surrounding this plant are enjoyment, letting yourself be touched, becoming soft, and discovering beauty for yourself.

Aphrodite's Anise Rings

You can serve this pastry without an ulterior motive of any kind, and you can use them as an offering as well.

You will need:

2 sticks plus 2 tbsp. butter

1¼ cup sugar

1 tsp. vanilla extract, or ground vanilla to taste

4 eggs

2 cups flour

3½ ounces ground hazelnuts (about 1⅓ cups)

2 tbsp. of ground anise

Gently warm the butter (not too hot or the egg you are about to add will congeal) and stir in the sugar and vanilla. Next, add two of the four eggs and keep stirring until it turns into a consistent mass. Take a sifter and slowly sift in some flour, then take turns stirring and sifting until the flour is mixed in completely. Knead in the ground hazelnuts and the ground anise and put the dough into the fridge for at least an hour. Do not skip this step or the dough will fall apart. Before you begin, heat the oven to 350 to 400 degrees. If you have a pastry bag, you can squeeze the dough onto a cookie sheet covered with parchment paper. I simply form small rolls by hand and shape it into rings. Separate the two remaining eggs and mix the yolks with a few drops of sugar water. It will give the pastry a nice color (but this isn't mandatory). Brush the cookies with it and bake them for fifteen minutes. Keep an eye on the cookies and check them occasionally to see if they are done (every oven is a little different).

Anise Schnapps

It would be easy to buy a bottle of Ouzo, but most herbal witches prefer to make their own. Here is a recipe for anise schnapps that can also be used for cooking and baking as a flavoring. You simply need a liter of neutral grain alcohol (vodka, corn whiskey, white whiskey, moonshine, etc.), about 7–9 ounces of anise seed (about two cups, give or take to desired intensity) and a clean container with an airtight seal.

Lightly crush the seeds in a mortar. (Do not use a kitchen appliance because it releases too many volatile oils that you want in the schnapps, not the machine.) Next, add the crushed anise seeds to the alcohol, seal the container and leave in in a warm place for a month, on the windowsill for example. Shake it occasionally when you walk by. Strain the seeds afterward, and your anise schnapps is done.

Basil

(Ocimum basilicum)

In cultures where it is known, basil is generally considered a lucky plant that wards off anything negative and enhances anything good. Since we mostly use it as a spice, many of us are unaware that it can do a lot more than pep up tomato sauce and pizzas.

Basil has a relaxing effect and is also a gentle aphrodisiac. It can be used during slightly depressed moods to lift the mood and reawaken the spirits of life. It further supports digestive health and general indisposition that is hard to localize. It can be used as a strengthening tonic and is also an excellent choice against nausea and motion sickness.

Magically, basil is used as a love potion and for general good luck. It can be found in many candle magic spells, as well as in magical waters, as a cleaning agent, and in herbal bouquets in folk magic.

Basil-Flavored Oil from Fresh Herbs

Basil oil tastes best when it is made from fresh basil. To avoid any molding of the water-based plant in the oil, the container must be kept in a warm place and cannot have an airtight seal. The neck of the container should be fairly wide. Pickling jars covered with a clean kitchen towel or a fine sieve are ideal. It must rest in a warm place. If streaks appear it is too cold and must be warmed until the oil is clear again (a hair dryer or heater can be helpful in this situation).

You can strain the oil after about two weeks and pour it into airtight containers. You will now have strongly aromatic basil oil; the kind dried basil could never yield. It can be used in the kitchen or for magical purposes.

Birch
(Betula spp.)

The birch tree holds the power of the moon and the sun. As the European ash was to the old Germans, and the oak tree is to us today, the birch tree was to the Siberian shamans a tree of thresholds and ultimately the tree of life itself. This concept can also be found in German-speaking regions. The traditional May tree was often a birch tree and I can recall from childhood a dancer decorated from head to toe in birch branches who would travel from house to house during Whitsuntide. He embodied springtime, danced in all the yards and received schnapps in every one of them, making his job a true challenge over the course of his visits.

In folk medicine the birch tree also holds a strong connection to spring and therefore to a sense of renewal, cleansing, and rejuvenation. A tea made from its leaves detoxes the body and cleanses the blood. Many natural pharmacies sell bottles of birch sap for purging purposes. As a bath additive, it gives new elasticity to the skin and gets rid of blemishes. Birch leaf has a cleansing and tonic effect on the kidneys and bladder and as such can be enjoyed as a tea or a bath in times of stress. Birch trees hold a soft energy full of light that can penetrate the foggiest veil and instill new confidence.

Generally, many old ideas are attached to trees. These are similarly understood worldwide, which is why magic practitioners—despite individual differences—can often communicate without words. One example is the image of the tree as a magical intermediary between Heaven and Earth, but also as the home of souls (often depicted as birds in those trees) that wish to be re-embodied. The image of people springing from the mythic world tree exists anywhere from Eastern Europe to West Africa. The tree is the symbolic home of a person before birth and after death. In my area we find this idea closely tied to elder trees. Lore and legend clearly depict it as an ancestral tree.

Sometimes the ideas shift to the mythical realm. Here the first humans step down onto earth from a magical tree. In the old traditions the (symbolic) birds also serve as the intermediaries between humans and the gods high up in the World Tree. The mythical arrival of the first humans on earth was even tied to a tree in the Bible—even if it was linked to negative omens. It was the Tree of Knowledge with its wondrous fruit.

Birch Leaf Bath

Take two handfuls of birch leaves (fresh or dried) and let them steep in cold water overnight in a big pot (with a lid). Next, warm the pot lightly. The temperature shouldn't get too hot. Under no circumstances should the liquid be brought to a boil. When the liquid is lukewarm, let it steep for fifteen minutes, then sift out the leaves and add the resulting liquid to a bath. Do not add anything else to the water, and soak in it for about twenty minutes. Do not towel off afterward, but let the water air dry on your skin.

Calendula

(Calendula officinalis)

With calendula we encounter our first "officinalis" plant. The epithet "officinalis" in a plant name means that the particular plant was available in an officine, the predecessor to our modern pharmacy. Beginning in the middle ages, the mostly itinerant herb peddlers often settled in cities and opened the officine. The "officinalis" plants are those plants that would be available in the pharmacy.

Calendula is an important healing plant for the skin. It is a mild cleanser with great effect in regard to skin infections (fungi, viruses, bacteria, and all of those ugly things they trigger) and was used to heal wounds in the old days. Today we see a doctor for serious wounds. Calendula can still help.

When a wound is no longer wet, calendula can aid the healing process and eases any tension on the tissue. It used to draw great appreciation during breast surgeries (and it is regaining attention today). Calendula is also an excellent helper after C-sections and all operations that leave a scar. You can begin by gently placing a clean cloth soaked in calendula tea on the area. You can also apply calendula salve around the wound. Its healing properties will reach the skin and the surrounding tissue. In addition, drink one to three cups of calendula tea a day. Once the wound has closed and simply has to heal, you can apply the salve directly to the affected area to facilitate healing and minimize tension to the scar.

Calendula salve is also much appreciated as a vein remedy, and it tightens the tissue. As a liver plant (it is slightly bitter) it can have a soothing effect during PMS. Be sparing with preparations containing the often-praised monk's pepper (Vitex agnus-castus, also called chasteberry), which did not get its name for nothing; monk's pepper was used to quench desire in the old days. That may not be your intended result. If you have to use it, use it during the second half of your cycle, not throughout the entire cycle.

Classic Calendula Salve

Different types of calendula creams can be found in any drug store, usually marketed for infants, but perhaps you feel like trying the classic recipe of our grandmothers. You will need fresh calendula. You can grow them yourself—make sure they are calendula, not the commonly confused marigolds (genus name Tagetes). You can even grow them on your windowsill. They should be harvested in full bloom in the late morning to let the dew evaporate, but before the plant is exhausted from the noontime heat.

Calculate two handfuls of blossoms to two and a half cups of pork lard (unsalted). You can also give a generous handful to a cup of pork lard if you do not want too much salve. It's okay if a few leaves get lost in the mix, as they hold similar healing powers. If you would rather not use animal fat you can use Shea butter or Vaseline instead. In this case you should make the salve using a bain-marie (double boiler), simmering for two hours. In my opinion, it's a little silly if a person who eats meat finds using lard unreasonable; why not utilize the whole animal?

Heat the lard in a pot, add the blossoms and stir them in well. Take the lard off the heat and let stand overnight, which will make it solidify again. Heat it again the next day, sift out the blossoms, and pour the calendula salve into a container.

Chamomile

(Matricaria chamomilla)

If we put folk medicine under the magnifying glass in regard to chamomile, it becomes difficult to find an ailment for which it does not at least offer some relief. Chamomile as matricaria (mother care) looks after mothers and their children. It helps with stomach problems and women's ailments, soothes the skin and relaxes the nerves. It is a good choice for relaxation because it belongs to the non-drowsy category of plants. Its calming effect is supportive when quitting bad habits, such as smoking. Many folk healers swear that nothing supports quitting smoking as well as chamomile tea does.

Chamomile was also considered *the* beauty treatment for skin and hair. Mucus membranes in the mouth, stomach, and intestines also benefit from it. People (not just blondes) often used to rinse out their hair with warm chamomile tea after shampooing and washed their faces in chamomile tea. You can also buy a chamomile tincture in the drug store and add it to water if you want a faster approach. Chamomile tincture can also be mixed into crèmes, lotions, shower gels, shampoos, and the like.

Emotionally, chamomile has a tension-releasing and cleansing effect. Those who are stressed and have a lot of irons in the fire will especially profit from its use. Do not hesitate to make some chamomile tea if you are under great strain personally or professionally.

I've been told by more than just one woman that their man unexpectedly became interested in them sensuously again after drinking the tea. Chamomile seems to have an aphrodisiac effect, especially on stressed men.

For pregnant women who have to be careful with healing plants, chamomile (but not Roman chamomile, a different species) and lady's mantle are recommended as a healing duo for all phases of life.

Chamomile as Incense

Many do not know that chamomile blossoms also make wonderful incense. They have an especially aromatic scent, cleanse rooms of all bad energies, and have a harmonizing and balancing effect.

Chamomile Steam Bath

In the case of vaginal yeast infections, you will rarely find a simpler treatment than a chamomile steam bath. All you will need is a heat-resistant bowl, chamomile tea or tincture, a big towel, and hot water.

Pour the hot water into the bowl along with a handful of chamomile blossoms or a few generous squirts of chamomile tincture. Next, kneel above the bowl for ten to fifteen minutes and place the towel like a tent around your legs in order to keep the steam contained.

The trick lies in the fact that chamomile in liquid form disinfects especially well, which means that a steam bath has a stronger effect than a warm compress or a douche would have, for example. At first glance a steam bath may seem inconvenient (after all, everything has to happen in a hurry these days), however, the desired result is often apparent after only one application—which takes less time than the trip to the pharmacy. If it has to be fast, do it right!

Chamomile Bath against Exhaustion

Not only does a chamomile bath give you beautiful skin, it is also refreshing when one is dog tired and hyped up at the same time. Those who have experienced stress over a prolonged period of time, faced too much work, big personal challenges, or simply the normal craziness of the everyday world will know this feeling. Even though one feels a leaden sense of exhaustion, one is filled with nervous tension and hyper at the same time. It goes without saying that you have to change something about the situation itself in this case. However, to help you unwind in the moment and to relax, a chamomile bath is excellent.

Take one to two handfuls of chamomile blossoms and pour about one and a half quarts of hot water over them. Next, seal the pot quickly with a tight-fitting lid and let the whole thing steep for fifteen minutes. Strain off the chamomile blossoms and add the stock to the bath water. Do not use additional bath supplements.

The quick version: Those who do not have the patience for this can take chamomile tincture to add a generous amount to the bath water (amount recommendations are on the package). Again, do not add bath supplements.

Bathe for about twenty minutes. Afterward, do not towel off if you can avoid it, but let the bath water air dry on the skin.

Cleavers (Sticky-Willy, Catchweed)
(Galium aparine)

Cleavers is one of the almost forgotten healing herbs, even though it has tremendous potential. Cleavers has a strong blood-cleansing effect and is used for acne as well as psoriasis and other reddening, itchy skin ailments. Generally, it works against anything that itches, even dandruff (treatments with lukewarm tea) or gum problems (gargle and rinse with the tea, then do not eat or drink anything for half an hour to let it seep in) as well as vaginal itching (rinses or compresses with soaked cloths). The wonderful thing about this plant is that it is very effective and at the same time very mild. Instead of fighting fire with fire, the "burn" is extinguished by gentle cooling.

It can be internally drunk as a tea or topically applied as mentioned above as a salve or a rinse. A tea cure with cleavers cleanses the body be it after a long bout of medication or as a strengthening tool after virus infections. Those who are constantly battling herpes, for example, should give cleavers a try for a change.

On the emotional level the herb has a cooling effect on feelings that tend to boil up. It refreshes the soul, has a relaxing effect and is also recommended as gentle support during sleep deprivation—even though it is non-drowsy. In times of stress you can also drink it as a relaxing tea during the day without a problem.

Cleavers can be found in the herbal pharmacy or you can pick it yourself. It grows as a weed in many damp areas. Put it in the oven at about 100–110 degrees in order to dry it. The herb will be done when it is dry enough to crack. No dampness should remain or it will mold easily.

My Family's Cleavers Salve

My family used and still uses this salve quite often whenever one of us has skin problems, especially during skin conditions that are scaly, itchy or leave the skin red. It calms and soothes the tissue and brings at least relief even in severe cases, sometimes even leads to a complete cure. It is also a good choice for cold sores. It stops them quickly and supports healing.

For the salve you will need around 9 ounces (1 ¼ cup or so) of Vaseline; as an alternative you can use Shea butter or other basic skin-safe ingredients that contain fats and have the consistency of a salve. (Unsalted lard was popular in the old days.) Add an ounce of dried cleavers to it (about a cup).

Melt the fat in a bain-marie (double boiler). As soon as it has reached liquid form, add the cleavers. Now let the bain-marie simmer for two hours (boil gently). You will have to keep adding water to the lower pot occasionally; in other words, keep an eye on the whole thing. Afterward sift off the herbs and fill clean containers with the salve.

The salve does not exactly have a spectacular scent. (I realized I should mention this after a friend looked at me aghast when he smelled it.) It is a pure salve without artificial scent additives. Many people are no longer familiar with this. It is about the effect in this case, not artificial wellness.

If you want, you can add a touch of essential oils to improve the scent, although I would personally never alter the salve. Not everything has to be prettied up. We should allow some things to remain real and gritty—in my opinion. It's fine if you see it differently.

Lavender(Lavandula angustifolia)

Lavender is primarily known as a sedative, and is used as such in the form of an essential oil in a scent lamp, in aromatherapy products, or as tea made from lavender blossoms. It is also effective against skin and nail fungi. It soothes the stomach, intestines, and gallbladder and can help you up during times of exhaustion. It is the best thing that can happen to you after a long stressful day at work. Even the pharmaceutical industry has caught on by now and has started advertising expensive lavender products.

You can do this in a much simpler and definitely cheaper way by drinking a cup of lavender blossom tea. As with all teas whose effect is based on their scent, make sure you cover the cup while it is steeping. Again, common sense should be used. Lavender is a strong healing herb. If the dosage is too high it can lead to dizziness. That does not mean that lavender is dangerous in any way, but herbs have a real effect similar to medication, which are not taken willy-nilly either. Emotionally, lavender has a supportive effect when it comes to relaxation. It can drag you out of the everyday and lends new strength to your nerves.

Lavender Applications

You can make a lavender pillow or fill ready-made sachets with lavender to protect the wardrobe and coat closet from moths. Little pouches like that are also wonderful next to the pillow as a gentle sleep aid. Simply knead it thoroughly before you go to bed to release the scent.

Since we are on the topic, lavender is a simple and non-poisonous remedy against ants in the household. Reading the warning labels on chemical ant repellants can be frightening—and somewhere there is a huge factory where the stuff is being mixed by the ton. There is a much easier and relaxing way to prevent ants, especially if you have children or pets in the home. First you have to clear away and lock up anything sweet that could attract the little crawlers. Next, find out where they are going and scatter lavender blossoms in their way. They act as a natural stop sign. I always mix in a few cloves or star-anise to make it more aromatic and—from the perspective of the ant—more sinister. Even the last stragglers are usually gone after two to three days and you can sweep up the whole thing. The three days of "lavender thresh" on the floor and the furniture is bearable and afterward you can rest with the good feeling that you didn't kill or poison anyone, including yourself. This is a fine, diplomatic solution on the level of scents.

Common and Wild Thyme ⊘
(Thymus spp.)

Both common and wild thyme (T. vulgaris and T. serpyllum) are used identically in folk medicine. Thyme is of great help during colds and persistent coughs. It breaks down mucus and ensures that you will get rid of a cold in a speedy fashion. Since it also loosens cramps, it is used for period pain, as well as a supportive aid in childbirth. Traditionally it is considered a protective plant that wards off any negative energy from mother and child following birth. It strengthens the spirits of both. Since it is an emmenagogue (an herb that encourages the period) in larger doses, it should not be used as a healing plant during pregnancy, but only when it is time.

Thyme is home to fairies. It was also known as the herb of Venus, who was considered to be the leader of the fairies as a female goddess in the old folk beliefs. She is similar to Holle with her small entourage. Thyme aids digestion, but also stimulates the metabolism. As such it is a good choice if one has a hangover or when trying to bring the body back to balance after taking strong medication. In Thuringia (and interestingly enough also in African American Hoodoo) it is also considered helpful when trying to gain wealth.

The great herbalist Maria Treben recommended thyme in cases of painful neuralgia, but also as support for paralysis, multiple sclerosis, rheumatism, and for recovery after strokes. It seems that it is also an herb for the hard times in life. We can sum it up simply: thyme invigorates and organizes the body.

Thyme Bath for Aching Limbs

To make a thyme bath, put on a big pot of water and bring it to a boil. Take the pot off the stove, add a cup of dried thyme, and seal the pot with a lid. Let it steep for fifteen minutes. Afterward you can strain out the herbs and add the resulting liquid to your bath water. Bathe for about twenty minutes and don't towel off. Rather, wrap up warmly in an old shirt and warm blankets and "keep steaming" a bit longer.

Cowslip ⊘
(Primula veris)

Cowslip is a fey plant. It's said magical fairy women holding keys to hidden treasures swarm around its blossoms. Isn't that a wonderful prospect!

In Germany cowslip is a protected plant (it is illegal to remove them from the wild). You can grow it yourself, though, or buy it from any herb merchant you trust. It unlocks the sinuses and opens the nose when mucus can't drain during colds. It is a first choice for ailments in this area.

Emotionally, cowslip has an opening and cleansing effect as well. It is known as a plant that lightens the heart during off moods or low spirits. As a non-drowsy plant, it can be used during the day and not just in the evenings.

Cowslip Syrup

This syrup is wonderful in mineral water, champagne, punch bowls, homemade ice cream, milk froth, coffee or however you can think of using it.

The base recipe is very simple. Take five cups sugar and one quart of water and bring both to a boil in a pot. Let the whole thing simmer until it has the consistency of syrup. It should be a little thicker than water. Take the pot off the stove and stir in two untreated lemons (cut into slices) and two handfuls of cowslip blossoms. Let the whole thing cool off under a closed lid. Then simply let the syrup stand in a cool space for three days (don't worry, the sugar conserves it). Afterward you can strain it and fill containers with it. Keep in the refrigerator.

Dandelion
(Taraxacum officinale)

Dandelion is certainly no weed. Its Latin name again contains the word "officinale," meaning it used to be a solid piece in any pharmacy in the old days. If only the gardeners and their poison sprayers knew what a treasure they had in front of them.

Dandelion is the quintessential plant for metabolism. It supports the liver and gallbladder, gently encourages the intestines, and can be helpful in cases of diabetes (discuss this with your doctor or health practitioner in this case). It helps against a loss of appetite (this used to be considered a problem rather than a desirable state) and has a stimulating effect on the body. If you have a hangover after a party, one to two cups of dandelion tea can help you set things right again.

Since dandelion has a positive influence on the liver, it automatically has a tonic effect on the entire body. The liver is our chemical factory. What is good for the liver is good for the entire body, which is why we can't fence in the effects of dandelion. It has an excellent effect on acne and unclean skin because it brings harmony and balances the metabolism.

Fresh dandelion juice can eliminate warts, which is well known. Emotionally, dandelion can help when someone has walked on your proverbial liver (a German expression for when someone bothers or peeves you) or when you are dealt a low blow and have to get back on your feet. It can also help in times of blockage—when you are stuck and can't really move forward and are thinking about things in an indecisive way. It will help you find a clear position, see the big picture. In this case it encourages your appetite figuratively; it creates a newfound appetite for life.

My Tried and True Acne Tea

Acne is not only a problem among teens. We could write a book about that in my family! Since I know from experience how much one suffers from it, it is especially important to me to pass this recipe along. One thing bcforc I start: don't expect miracles overnight and keep with it for a while, even if you suffer setbacks. Herbs do not work like manufactured chemicals! For support, use masks with healing clay, which you can find in some drug stores and many health food stores—look for French green clay, bentonite clay, fuller's earth, kaolin clay, etc. In acute phases apply the clay directly to the affected area every two days. In calm phases apply every one to two weeks to the entire face or the affected area. Don't make any excuses like "I don't have time for this kind of thing." You can find time to sit in front of the TV at night. So, sit in front of it for fifteen minutes with healing clay on your face.

The essential ingredients for my acne tea are dandelion and stinging nettle; add other skin soothing plants you have available such as chamomile, walnut leaves, horsetail, cleavers, pansies, birch leaves, calendula, or elder blossoms. You can add pieces of apple, mint, lemongrass or similar plants for the benefit of taste. Drink the tea two to three times a day during acute phases. In calm phases only drink it occasionally. It shouldn't be taken continuously in the long term because the body will get used to it and stop reacting as well. Nothing says you can't drink this tea for two to three weeks at a time. It just shouldn't be two to three months at a time.

You can also change the ingredients in a variety of ways … a little bit of this one time, another plant a different time. I mix one cup of dandelion and stinging nettle each and add the rest of the plants by feeling until I have filled a tea tin.

If your skin problems are related to your cycle, meaning if you have premenstrual acne, add lady's mantle and yarrow to it. To prevent letting it get too muddled I would suggest in this case: lady's mantle, yarrow, stinging nettle and dandelion and not a whole lot else. For best results drink the tea from the middle of your cycle to your period. As soon as you feel the skin calming down you can simply drink it when you feel like it. In addition to its skin cleansing effect, it is also invigorating and relaxing and soothes the liver due to its positive effect on our inner chemical factory.

Elder

(Sambucus nigra)

Elder is also known as lilac in Northern Germany today, although they are different plants. The botanical diagram of its blossoms has symbolic power: the threefold goddess is in the center, surrounded by a pentagram. This is how it can be read.

In certain regions men still tip their hats to an elder bush today. It was considered a spirit tree and still is. Slavic people used it as a sacrificial place.

In many regions elder is a significant part of the household, was closely tied to the family, and was further considered an oracle. People worried that their farm was in jeopardy or expected a death in the family if the bush shriveled up. A baby's first bath was drawn under the elder bush in order to let it see the new citizen of earth.

In addition, elder bushes were supposed to protect the home from lightning strikes, fires, black magic, as well as poisonous envy. It was connected to Mother Holle and later to the Virgin Mary. Where the transition to Christianity was less than smooth, dark stories grew around the elder like tendrils. In these cases, helpful house spirits, fairies, elves, and goddesses suddenly turned into sinister beings that wished to do all kinds of evil things to passersby or anyone who slept under an elder bush. But why would any reputable house have a house elder if it attracted bad fortune? That makes no sense at all. However, a few precautions did exist: babies were not supposed to sleep in cribs made from elder wood because a bush that is so closely associated with fairies holds much of their energy. This affects the little ones more than adults and it could be too much for them.

In folk medicine, elderberries in juice form or prepared as a tea is well known for its healing effects against colds, fever, and in the treatment of bladder and kidney problems. However, use only ripe berries, and boil it if you are making it yourself; it is quite poisonous when uncooked, causing diarrhea and vomiting. Elder is a good supportive choice for sinusitis and coughs.

Modern herbal science broadened this spectrum to include elder as a calming, grounding plant in times of stress and exhaustion. It can further serve to cure headaches—without any side effects. In terms of relaxation, the flowers are primarily used to make a syrup or tea. The tea made from elderflowers can also be used as a compress or for gentle topical application in the case of rash or skin problems. It is very mild and tends to calm the tissue instead of aggravating it. As such, it is certainly worth a try.

Especially in regard to skin problems it can take a while until one discovers "their" plant(s). You shouldn't throw in the towel if it does not work right away. What do you have to lose?

Most plants can be wonderfully brewed as an herbal tea if they don't seem to work on the skin. When you have found your favorites, you will have affordable helpers (in comparison with most medications) without side effects worth mentioning. At the very least they will serve as a solid first aid.

Although herbs may not always be able to replace a physician, they will give you the good feeling of being able to do something for yourself as well; knowing you are not completely reliant on others, but know how to help yourself.

Emotionally, elder is a big help after one has experienced deep wounds or shocking, overwhelming situations. When someone has died, when a goodbye was painful, after you have been fired at work, experienced a broken friendship that meant a lot to you—all of the things that affect the heart—elder can help surmount these issues. Tea made from elderflower blossoms especially helps in this case. You can also add elder syrup to your tea. Elder will work for you of its own accord.

Elderflower Syrup

This syrup is very easy to make.

You will need:

15 to 20 fresh umbels *or* 1 cup of dried elder blossoms

1 quart of water

10 cups sugar

3 untreated lemons or limes

If you are using the fresh umbels, which are more aromatic than dried blossoms, place them on a piece of paper first to allow all small critters to crawl away. Afterward, cut the flowers in a way that leaves as little stem as possible and place it into a wide glass or a bowl. Pour the lukewarm water over it next, add the sugar, cut the lemons or limes into eighths and add them as well. Stir the whole thing well to allow the sugar (the conserving ingredient) to dissolve completely.

Let this mixture stand at room temperature for two to three days and run it through a sieve (preferably a cloth) afterward. It can be bottled or placed in kitchen containers with a good seal. The syrup is not very perishable due to the sugar, although it often does not last long simply because it is so tasty.

You can also freeze the syrup. Since it went through cold processing the fine aroma of the blossoms does not fade, which would quickly be the case if we were to boil it.

English Walnut Leaves

(Juglans regia)

In their fresh state, English walnut leaves have an unrivaled sweet, herbal, and aromatic odor. In natural medicine they are used for rinses, compresses, and baths whenever the skin suffers. In cases of acne, but also for itchy skin, rashes, and scaly skin, make a tea and cool it to lukewarm. Place a tea-soaked cotton cloth on the affected area for fifteen minutes.

To make an English walnut leaf bath, put on a big pot of water, add a small cup of the leaves, bring to a boil, then take it off the stove. Let it cool, sift out the leaves, and add the liquid to the bath water.

English walnut leaf tea can also help in cases of internal infections. It cleanses the digestive tract and lends new strength from within. It is also cleansing for the skin since it cleanses the intestines. The rule in herbal medicine is if something is wrong externally (meaning on the skin), something is also wrong internally, which is why it is pointless to treat only the external symptoms. The body is a whole organism.

Due to the rich concentration of tannins they contain, walnut leaves have an astringent effect and help against fungi and bacteria. A rinse with lukewarm walnut leaf tea after shampooing can also be very effective against dandruff, a scabby head, as well as an itchy scalp. Don't do this on very light hair, however, since it can lead to slightly darkening results.

Ever since the old days, walnuts have been considered symbols of general fertility, like all nuts (the well protected nut encased in a tight shell is reminiscent of the stomach of a pregnant woman). The belief still exists today that the year following a rich walnut harvest will bring the births of many children. Is this connected to the ingredients contained in the nut? A woman who wishes for a child can try to eat a few nuts on a regular basis. It certainly can't hurt.

Walnut Schnapps for the Skin

Take a sealable jar (pickling jars are ideal) and add chopped fresh green walnut pieces (in their green shell before they ripen). Pour a clear grain alcohol over them such as vodka or moonshine and let the whole thing stand for two weeks. The liquid will darken considerably over this time. Afterward, sift off the liquid and fill containers with the resulting walnut schnapps. Diluted with water, it is ideal for compresses and rinses to treat acne, unclear skin, skin infections and the like. Add a generous squirt to the wash water and wash your face with it. Do this without adding soap or anything else, but simply use water and schnapps.

Generally, this is an important ground rule: many skin problems disappear on their own if you forego strong detergents in soap and body wash. Many dermatologists confirm this; if the skin is degreased too much its natural balance is disturbed, making it vulnerable to microbes. Alternatively, you can also use healing clay, or a mild face-cleansing milk as a body wash. These products have a cleansing effect without throwing the skin off balance. Skin problems often clear up when we switch to baby shampoo or baby shower gels. Those who do not have a problem have no reason to switch, but if you have dry or sensitive skin, give it a try. There is no overall cure, but it is remarkable that we aggressively remove oil from the skin with shower gels and so on and then try to get it halfway fit again with lotions and creams. The skin can take good care of itself if we let it. Cleanliness is important, but our selection of products is crucial in order to feel fresh without burdening the skin with additional chemicals, regardless of how "moisturizing," "gentle," or "nurturing" the advertisements make them out to be.

This is also true for the face. If at all possible, don't use face creams every day. Of course, advertisements try to convince us that we will look like a collapsed soufflé within a short amount of time if we don't use them daily (and possibly even nightly as well). After all, the big companies want to make money and they do make huge profits. However, too much care can make the skin lazy and can irritate it and even damage it in the worst-case scenario. Many of us seem to forget that the skin is an organ. After all, we wouldn't glue our eyes, heart, or kidneys shut. This comparison is a stretch, of course, but we should be aware that the skin is first and foremost a natural organ that wants to (and can) do its job.

The best anti-wrinkle treatment is having healthy blood flow through movement, and the blood needs quality nutrients that are absorbed through our diet. Once again, we're looking at the body as a whole. When the mirror instills fear in you because your skin looks pale or flat, or you have circles under your eyes that rival those of a panda bear, you should be grateful that your body is sending you signals. Something is wrong. Everyone has a bad day now and then, but when this turns into a permanent state you have to come clean with yourself and think about what you can change overall.

Hawthorn

(Crataegus spp.)

Hawthorn is fairly well known as a heart-strengthening plant. In addition to teas, we can also take advantage of convenient ready-made concoctions in the form of pills or capsules, which is a good idea if you can't make peace with its slightly musty taste.

In the healing science of the Travelers as well as in Alpine regions, people know that the heart-strengthening effect is ultimately emotional in nature. Hawthorn helps all those with a broken heart, a heavy heart, or otherwise suffer from heart pains. Folk sayings are often very specific in their terminology. Next to linden blossoms, hawthorn is plant helper number one whenever you suffer from love sickness.

Hawthorn stabilizes the metabolism. It can balance out blood pressure that is too low, but too high as well, which means that it ensures the correct measure. The plant has to be consumed on a regular basis in order to do this. As such, hawthorn is among the plants one should use as a longer cure, since it builds its effects gradually. It is also suitable for problems that are not physical, but gnaw at you subconsciously. Let's put it this way: it cleanses the heart, but does not clean up in one swipe. It conscientiously tackles one corner after another.

The emotionally relaxing (non-drowsy) effects of hawthorn can help with sleep troubles as well, especially when you lie in bed ruminating and can't seem to find closure to your day.

In the old days hawthorn was among the repelling plants for magic spells and at the same time was home to good fairies.

When a child has trouble sleeping or nightmares, a small bundle of hawthorn in the bed serves as protection (of course adults can also give this a try). It is best to search for it together. Kids love activities like this and it gives them the good feeling that they are not defenseless and vulnerable, but that there is something they can do themselves. When a baby cries too much or is easily frightened hawthorn bunches can also be used. Our ancestors saw crying and fear as the influence of evil fairies. I don't think we should fall back into the past without reflecting, but a small bunch of hawthorn can't hurt and maybe it will help.

Those who were in need of luck would braid a few hairs and/or pieces of material from a worn piece of clothing into a hawthorn bush as a sign to the fairies that they needed help.

Bunches of Hawthorn

All you need to do in order to find hawthorn is to simply open your eyes. Sometimes it even grows in a park right in the center of the city. During its blooming time from May to June you can immediately identify it by its slightly musty aroma. It smells of a little almond, a little rose (it is in the family of rose plants), and a little carrion. You look at the bush and think: oh, how beautiful. You get closer to it and your nose says, "Oh no!" That's how you can tell that you are right. Cut off a bundle of the twigs for yourself. It does not have to be much. Folk magic often used little twigs the length of a finger when it came to bringing the good healing powers of the trees into the home. Tie your bunch with a white ribbon or twine and hang it over your bed or over the bed of your child. If this is not an option because it is inconvenient or you simply don't want to explain it to others, you can place the bunch under the mattress or (even more directly) work it into the stuffing of the pillow by creating an opening and sewing it shut again.

Let's assume that in spite of all your efforts you have not been able to find any hawthorn or have not had time or patience to look. This happens. In this case buy yourself some dried hawthorn, preferably a mixture of leaves and blossoms, and fill a small white sachet with them. About as much as you can easily close your hand around. Seal the bag with a white ribbon and proceed as described above.

Horsetail

(Equisetum arvense)

Horsetail is the herb for skin, hair, and nails overall; rich in minerals, it supports hair growth and contains plenty of silicic acid. For centuries it has been described as a Saturn plant due to its benefit to bones and joints. It doesn't work overnight, but builds up over a long-term period. This is important to know when working with plants. It can also be applied as a supportive aid in cases of osteoporosis, gout, sports-related injuries, or spinal disc problems.

In addition, it has a detoxing and draining effect. In the old days people used to say that horsehair "takes pressure off the kidneys," which meant that it was emotionally relaxing. (If something goes to your kidneys, horsetail will flush it from the body.) Horsetail restores your balance when you feel frayed or unraveled and are stuck in situations in which you are unsure what to tackle first.

It helps ward off nervousness, fear, and symptoms of stress. Even though horsetail can't boast of a relaxing scent or a charming aroma, it is a plant good for the soul because it relieves pressure.

Application

You can grind horsehair into a powder or buy it in powder form and consume half a teaspoon occasionally. If you want to drink it as a tea, I recommend boiling the plant thoroughly. Simply pouring boiling water over it does not release the active ingredients as well as boiling it well does. Let a teaspoon per cup boil over low heat for about ten to fifteen minutes. You will see the difference in the liquid as it will turn a strong green color. Drink the tea as a cure for best results—one cup three times a day. Since most of us do not have time to boil tea for fifteen minutes three times a day (even though it would be a great relaxation activity), a thermos is a good alternative. They make small models that are convenient to carry with you. You simply have to know how to help yourself.

Lady's Mantle and Yarrow

(Alchemilla vulgaris and Achillea millefolium)

Even though these plants are very different I would like to introduce them together, since a combination of the two constitutes *the* dream team against female problems of any kind. They strengthen the feminine in body, mind, and spirit. Lady's mantle has a gentle and protective effect, while yarrow is much stronger, and its bitter components bring harmony.

Both plants can be used individually or mixed one to one. They are excellent helpers when it comes to any inner tension before the period (especially lady's mantle) as well as menstrual ailments. They also support pregnancy. They further soothe the hormonal transition into puberty and menopause. Following surgeries to the abdomen they help stabilize and help the body regain its equilibrium. I like to mix the tea with a little green jasmine tea. It tastes better that way and it leaves me with a stimulating beverage for the day.

A compress made from lady's mantle, yarrow, and chamomile can reduce painful swelling of the breasts before menstruation or during pregnancy.

Due to the bitter substance contained in yarrow, it is one of the more blood cleansing herbs and helps with premenstrual acne as well. It was often given in the form of a tea to children with a tendency to wet the bed. Lady's mantle is among the plants that can balance and trigger hormones, specifically the luteinizing hormone. Women that tend to have vaginal spotting before their period, have very short cycles, or worry that they can't carry an embryo to term due to a weakness of the corpus luteum should try a cure with lady's mantle if their doctor does not have an objection to it.

When it comes to female issues, emotional causes are often considered, which is certainly not wrong. However, we have to consider this: we live surrounded by substances that act similarly to hormones, specifically in cosmetics, synthetic perfumes, and everyday plastic items. The remnants of hormones given in pill form or in medication make their way into the water cycle, which can then enter our bodies.

I often wondered why I could find tips pertaining to menstrual pain, but no advice against the premenstrual tensions that plague so many women today in old books on herbs. I cannot prove a connection, but it certainly stands out. We can't always pretend that one gender should be to blame for all of this—women are so sensitive after all—or constantly has emotional problems. The entire community has a problem when something like this happens. We have to look at the whole picture instead of letting one individual take the blame for her environment.

As far as premenstrual syndrome (PMS) goes, the term syndrome alone does not have a pleasant connotation. It automatically conjures up the thought of serious illnesses. I myself use this term at several points in this book so that everyone will know what I am talking about, but certainly not because I enjoy it. How is a woman supposed to find her true power under this figurative sword of Damocles? Especially since, at a certain age, menstruation is simply a sign of physical health. No "time of the month" would mean no fertility and thus no life. Look around: every single person you see is here because a woman said yes and carried the child to term.

The negative views on menstruation and the days that precede it prevail primarily in Western cultures. In other cultures, people speak of HSC, high spiritual consciousness. From the sorceresses of West Africa to the shamans of Siberia the time starting one week before menstruation to the end of the period is considered the strongest spiritual phase of a woman. It is the time in which no one can fool a woman because she can tell exactly what people are really thinking. What we label as mood swings or an imbalance, other cultures consider a sign of incorruptibility and time for the establishment of the truth. There they believe that if you want to solve a problem, wait for this time of the month because the solution will come to you more easily. Women are described as more radiant and they have a magical charm during this time. Many taboos about menstruation were created to suppress the power of women. Her blessing as well as her curse is especially strong during this time because she is closer to otherworldly things.

Let's return to lady's mantle and yarrow. Here are a few suggestions for their use.

Women's Tea

Before menstruation a tea made from equal parts yarrow and lady's mantle is ideal. Drink at least one cup twice a day, for breakfast and in the evenings for example. If you suffer from bloating, drink the tea throughout the entire second half of your cycle (starting at the beginning of ovulation) and add birch leaves and stinging nettle to the mix (all equal parts, meaning the same amount from each of the four herbs).

Period Tea

If you suffer from a heavy or painful menstrual period, mix yarrow and capsella (shepherd's purse) one to one and add anise seeds (as much as you like). This mixture reduces excessive blood flow and brings harmony to the body.

Menopause Tea

Mix equal parts lady's mantle, yarrow, and lemon balm and fix yourself a tea as often as you like. It has a calming effect on the hormone system and helps prevent hot flashes. It does not have to be drunk every day, but the ritual should happen on a regular basis for it to act. Add a little bit of sage to the tea if you tend to break out in sweats (please heed the information pertaining to sage). Washing with sage or spraying cool sage tea from a spray bottle, like a body spray, eases ailments and feels good. If you prefer to use essential sage oil because you find it more practical, you shouldn't. This should only be used in a scent lamp and even then not around pregnant women or people who suffer from high blood pressure. It is okay in tea form, but the essential oil of sage is so strong that it can lead to side effects.

Essential oils are never found in nature in the high concentrations we are familiar with out of the bottle. In nature they are embedded in the whole plant rather than concentrated. Some oils are completely harmless and can even be ingested; however, this does not apply to all of them. This should be considered in advance.

Chest Compresses

Those who suffer from painfully swollen breasts before their period or during pregnancy can try this compress: prepare a tea from yarrow, chamomile, and lady's mantle (equal parts) and soak a white cloth in it. Take care to make sure the liquid is lukewarm and not too hot. Put the cloth on your breasts as wet as possible and put on one or two old shirts over it to allow for a humid environment. Let the whole thing seep in for about fifteen minutes (while watching TV at night perhaps). If you like, you can do it longer, or spray or dab your chest with rose water afterward. This is not mandatory, but a treat.

Joint Salve

One thing that is barely known today: people used to put tremendous trust in yarrow when it came to healing joint and back pain. Common folk could conveniently purchase this medicine at the side of the road. Its effects are apparent.

You will need one to two handfuls of fresh yarrow (just eyeball it). Place them on a white sheet of paper to allow any small critters that may still live in them to escape. Yarrow especially has many small friends, and no one wants to cook them into a salve.

When everyone has crawled out, heat about two cups of clarified butter to liquid form (directly in the pot without a bain-marie) and add the fresh yarrow to it. Take it off the stove and let it cool afterward until the butter has hardened again. This will take a few hours. Give it time. You can also let it cool overnight. Afterward heat the clarified butter up again until it reaches liquid form. Sift off the yarrow contained therein. The resulting salve now simply has to be packaged.

Linden Blossoms

(Tilia spp.)

Linden blossoms put out a rich sweet aroma and have a calming and relaxing effect when made into a tea. They are excellent during times of sleep deprivation and warm the soul in cold times. Those who suffer from high blood pressure can use linden blossoms as a supportive aid—after consulting with your physician, of course.

If you are looking to use an herb against a broken heart, consider linden blossoms. They strengthen from the inside out and get rid of bitterness and tension.

The linden tree is a holy tree, similar to the oak tree. Many villages have a village linden tree in their central square. It is not rare that you will find a bench to rest underneath it. People used to dance and celebrate under linden trees, but that is not all. Bast fiber from linden trees was used to make clothing, bags, ropes, and household items like mats in the old days. We still find the linden name in the names of towns today. My beloved Leipzig was derived from Lipsk, the place of lindens.

Linden Blossom Tea with Honey

This recipe is extremely simple and very effective in times of stress, when you face sorrow or the whole world seems to be crashing down on you. Boil a cup of tea from one teaspoon of linden blossoms in a cup, let it steep covered for ten minutes and add the honey. Stir it in and drink it sip for sip. Enjoy the tea. Make time for it even if it is only for fifteen minutes. Be present for it. Even *how* we do things like that contributes to its positive effect.

Mint

(Mentha spp.)

Mint is a cooling plant through and through. It helps during all "hot" imbalances such as fever and infections. It also helps in another sense whenever you feel you are running hot and need to cool off—to maintain the proverbial cool head. It is an excellent helper especially for those who work a lot and people affected by stress (of course this has to be turned off or balanced out—mint alone can't shoulder all of that).

In the ninth century, Strabo wrote, "If anyone claims to know all the powers, types, and names of mint, they may as well claim to know how many fish swim in the Red Sea or how many sparks Vulcanus, the melting-god of Lemnos, sends into the air over Mt. Aetna." What can you add to that? Mint is *the* healing plant against the small everyday things that leave us indisposed. It ranges from the invigorating mint lozenge to the drop of mint oil on the scalp or the neck to lessen tension, headaches, or even mosquito bites. Mint has a calming effect on digestion and was used in wealth magic, perhaps because the plant grows so prolifically wherever it sprouts.

Mint Oil

Add essential oil of mint to a carrier oil (unscented baby oil, jojoba oil, almond oil, sunflower oil—whatever you like). Try the dosage yourself. The whole thing also depends on the kind of mint you use. Peppermint oil is much stronger than oil made from spearmint or bergamot mint. Everyone reacts differently to it as well. Some people can't get enough of it and others only need a touch of it, anything else is too intense. But overall, do not use more than ten percent essential mint oil to the base oil. However, like I said, it is up to the individual to decide. Your nose has the final say.

You can use the homemade mint oil to dab your temples and your neck when you have a headache or stress. It has a soothing effect during colds and will help you regain your breathing. It revives one's spirits during fits of nausea. It cools insect bites and is invigorating while stimulating powers of concentration. We can truly say that if you have chamomile and mint in the house, you are well equipped to deal with anything that could leave you indisposed in your everyday life.

Mugwort ⊘

(Artemisia vulgaris)

Mugwort is primarily known as a plant that supports digestive health and is used for the Christmas goose, a German tradition. Its bitter components bring harmony to the body and stimulate the female cycle, which is why mugwort is among the herbs pregnant women should avoid.

Mugwort was able to do even more for our ancestors. It was said it could drive sickness spirits—imagined as worms and small snakes—from the body. As a side note, the god Odin supposedly overcame the Lindworm with the help of this plant.

Mugwort was also used in oracles and séances with ghosts in order to learn things from them and to basically force them to give up the desired information. Mugwort keeps "worms" of all kinds at bay. Just like St. John's wort this plant was preferably picked at the time of the summer solstice and used as preventative magic against illness in solstice wreaths. In addition, it was supposed to ward off lightning strikes and any bewitching. It was hung around the house for this purpose and often used as a protective ingredient in magic.

This plant, whose aroma is strong and herbal, holds an ancient, wise energy that does not put up with any nonsense, but focuses on what is essential. However, mugwort has a connection to love and the magic of love in addition to its strong spiritual vein. It was supposed to attract a partner and was often worn by widows who were looking to begin a second marriage.

Physically, mugwort has an overall harmonizing and strengthening effect. The image of something that serves as a remedy for worms is not necessarily false, you simply have to know how to classify it. Drink one cup of tea daily for one to two weeks for a short mugwort cure (one teaspoon dried herbs, steep for ten minutes). It can work wonders in times of stress.

The Magical Mugwort Belt

For a mugwort belt, which should ideally be fashioned on the feast day of John the Baptist (June 24) or shortly before that on the summer solstice (June 22). You will need red cloth and fresh mugwort. The belt does not have to be a handicraft masterpiece, since it will eventually be burned or given to a flowing body of water. Anyone can make it.

Cut a strip of cloth about four inches wide and long enough that you will comfortably be able to fit through it with your whole body if you lay it out in a circle. Think about a tight hula-hoop ring and add a few centimeters for the knot.

Place a moderate amount of fresh mugwort in the center of the cloth strip. Roll the cloth tight around the mugwort. You should have enough width in the cloth to completely wrap the herb (or use less mugwort). Then you can close the belt with basting stitches or wrap a band or ribbon around it.

Knot up the belt and come up with a small ceremony to use it. This does not have to be anything grandiose. All that matters is that it has a personal meaning to you.

Next, pull the belt across your body from head to toe. The main idea is that the mugwort rides across the whole body like a scanner and soaks up all of the negative energy. Step out of the belt and toss it into a fire or a river. This should happen immediately, so I recommend performing the ritual by a fire or a river in order to throw the belt into it instantly. After all, you do not want evil to have the chance to crawl back out of the mugwort and return.

This ritual is reminiscent of the trees that were split in order to pull the sick person through or of the stones with large holes through which people were similarly pulled to rid them of their illnesses. This goes back to the "drawing through" technique of removing illnesses and negative energies.

You can use this belt all year long whenever you are faced with a big streak of bad luck and everything seems to go wrong. If worse comes to worse, use dried mugwort in order to ward off anything evil and to cleanse yourself of it.

Oak ⊘

(Quercus spp.)

The oak is often considered a masculine tree. In Northern Germany, however, it is often referred to as the "gode olle," the good old lady. This puts it in the same category as the elder tree. Folk beliefs of many regions hold that it's connected to lightning, thunderstorms, and the associated nature spirits and gods such as Jupiter, Taranis, or Donar.

Alongside elder, spruce, and willow, oak joins to form the "magical four" in respect to the tying on of illnesses. These kinds of trees are most popular for this purpose in the old folk beliefs.

Oak and linden trees shared the position of court or village trees. In many villages, one of these trees is "the" tree and often surrounded by a bench to this day. What serves as a nice place to have a chat today was a courtroom in the old days.

The oak tree stands for luck, strength and energy. Our ancestors must have noticed its goal oriented, straight growth early on. Acorns were considered good luck amulets in regard to wealth and prosperity. They can still be used as such today, although there used to be a very concrete reason for this tradition: people used to drive pigs into oak woods in order to fatten them. The faith in the power of the oak was so strong that Christian missionaries would actually cut them down do destroy the sacred place of the "heathens." Conversion sometimes happened in more peaceful terms when oak trees were decorated with pictures of the Virgin Mary and Christ and thus incorporated into the cult.

Oak bark is a popular home remedy for skin problems. The natural tannins contained in the bark rid the skin of fungi and bacteria and help stabilize the skin's equilibrium. Oak bark can also be used on the "inner skin" in the form of a tea to balance the intestinal tract, among other things. Oak bark has a strengthening effect whether it is used as incense or tea. It is one of the best plant allies you can wish for whenever you have to weather a storm.

Oak Bark Tea

Add about one teaspoon of oak bark to two cups of water. Bring the mixture to a boil and steep for fifteen minutes.

You can spread out drinking this tea over the entire day or take it with you in a thermos. It has a cleansing effect and brings harmony to the body, especially to the intestines and digestion and the influence these have over the entire body. This tea should be used as a cure and not be consumed over a time period longer than two weeks.

Oak Bark Stock

Take the biggest pot you own and fill it with water. Add about one cup of oak bark. Bring the water to a boil and let it steep for fifteen minutes just like the tea described above. Siphon off the liquid and add it to a bath. Do not add any additional bath ingredients and bathe for about twenty minutes. Do not dry off with a towel, but let the water air dry on your skin.

You can use oak bark stock for skin problems of any kind. It is very gentle on account of the tannins. It soothes and eases, and essentially works as a gentle bludgeon because despite all of this it is extremely effective. You can also use this bath when you are feeling somewhat less than thick-skinned and need a bit of strengthening.

Oregano/Marjoram

(Origanum spp.)

Oregano (*Origanum vulgare*) is also called wild marjoram, but you can also use regular marjoram (*Origanum majorana*)—it stays in the (plant) family. It is considered antispasmodic and can be helpful during menstruation, which it also supports. Marjoram loosens cramps both physically and emotionally. It strengthens the back and reminds us of the strength we often possess without knowing we do. The science of plant healing refers to this as mood lifting. In the old days people used to say that it cures melancholy. An old epithet of marjoram is "light-hearted," which speaks for itself.

In the past, marjoram was often worked into salves in order to loosen tired or tense muscles. This is a useful field, in which it is still widely used today. Most people know marjoram as an herb that supports digestion today, although it meant much more to our ancestors. It belonged to those magical herbs that were supposed to ward off all evil and as such it was also used against sickness spirits. Brides used to wear it in a shoe and it was often mixed into bridal bouquets, which used to be more than simply decoration. They looked more like protective herbal shrubs that were meant to bring good luck. Burned as incense, marjoram has been famous for driving out negative energy since ancient times.

Dill with oregano and/or marjoram was considered a powerful combination. Hence the old spell: "I have dost (oregano), I have dill, XY does what I will (want)." This combination was often used against evil intentions, meaning it is an active magical formula that is supposed to stop others from evildoing. It has an incredibly focused energy, which makes it a wonderful tool for clearing thoughts.

Mood Lifting Incense Mix

Mix up a little marjoram, mint, St. John's wort, rosemary, lavender and a bit of aromatic resin such as pine, copal, mastic or elemi according to taste and preference (the whole thing should give off a fresh scent). Light this mixture whenever it pleases you. During tough times you can use it in the bedroom at bedtime. Afterward air the room out with windows wide open for five to ten minutes, and go to bed.

Sage
(Salvia officinalis)

Sage is among the best Mediterranean immigrants that found their way into our domestic herbal pharmacy via monastic gardens. Sage gets its name from the Latin word salvare, which means to heal.

Sage was and still is one of the great healing plants. However, like all remedies with strong healing powers, you want to use it with caution because sage contains thujone. It is not a suitable healing herb for pregnant women. Everyone else should remember not to consume more than four to six leaves a day and even that should not be done continuously. You essentially just have to listen to your gut; you will begin to feel nauseous fairly quickly if you take too much sage.

Taken in moderation, it is a wonderful healing remedy against colds, especially coughs and a scratchy throat—and thus the perfect herb for singers. I once had to smirk during a concert when the singer paused to tell the audience between songs she had to take a quick sip of sage tea. Sage also stimulates the brain and offers support in times of learning, during tests or strenuous tasks.

Sage tea is also a good choice for toothaches due to its disinfecting qualities. However, for infections along the gumline, a good old myrrh tincture can't be beaten. You can still find it in many pharmacies and in a few drug stores as well.

Sage can battle bacteria as well as viruses. As a wash or in (foot) baths it stops excessive sweating. It is recommended that you drink tea as well during a cure like this.

Sage Incense

Dried sage is among the most popular incense herbs and is itself combustible: you will not need any charcoal tabs or a teapot warmer to keep it smoking. Due to its slightly wooly consistency it is enough to briefly light it, then blow it out. It will die out on its own. You can also mix it with other herbs that will burn out with it. You simply have to experiment with which mix proportions are right for you.

Since sage smoke has an intense scent, you don't need to use much of it indoors. It is supportive during study and mental work of all kinds, clears rooms of all negative energy, and emits great healing powers.

If someone has been sick in the household the living quarters should be completely cleared with sage smoke. Afterward open the windows to let the smoke and all negative energies escape. I usually mix it with rosemary and aromatic resins such as copal or elemi, since sage smoke alone has too much of a smoky aroma for me. Do whatever best suits you. You can experiment with mixing and matching until it rounds out nicely for you.

Stinging Nettle/Common Nettle
(Urtica dioica)

The stinging nettle can undoubtedly be considered our greatest healing plant next to chamomile. It is an excellent strengthening remedy that cleanses and builds up the organism.

I highly recommend a springtime cure with nettle leaf tea. To do this you will simply have to drink one to three cups of stinging nettle tea daily over a two- to four-week time period. It energizes the metabolism and rejuvenates. Nettles can be used all year round, however—whenever you feel exhausted overall or are battling small infections. This makes it very attractive for people who play sports or otherwise wish for more spunk in life, especially in sensual terms. Stinging nettle seeds are still considered a lust ingredient. They are sometimes found in old love potions.

Besides its strong effects in the broad sense, nettle also has a few fields of specialization as well. It is a wonderful support in times of bladder and kidney ailments, for example. Beginning bladder infections can be brought under control with merely two or three cups of its tea without having to resort to chemical weapons. As a skin-hair-nail plant it additionally supports clean, fresh skin as well as nail and hair growth. As a hair growth remedy, it can be used as a hair tonic in addition to tea.

Stinging nettles were further used as a strengthening herb for bleeding after childbirth and used during heavy menstrual bleeding to bring the body back to harmony. It is an excellent tonic after surgeries as something that will help you get back on your feet. Another thing many people no longer consider today: the nettle has a close connection with the production of fabric and as such to many myths that have anything to do with spinning, weaving, and sewing—this also links it to the three spinners and the three goddesses of fate.

In old folk tales shirts made of nettles often make the heroes and heroines invincible or break an evil spell. These days it is hard to buy true nettle cloth. Most nettle fabrics today are made of cotton.

On an emotional level, nettle leaf has a strengthening and balancing effect. However, it generally tends to work through the body in the sense that strengthening the body ultimately has a positive effect on the soul.

It was considered good luck to eat stinging nettle soup on Holy Thursday, the Thursday before Easter, also called Maundy Thursday. This was meant to ensure that money did not run out in the coming year. The same belief was practiced on New Year's Day in other regions.

Holding one stinging nettle leaf for each finger in your hand was said to instill courage and fearlessness. As a Mars plant (due to the fact it burns) it was believed to protect against evil fairies and unruly nature spirits (our ancestors were aware that not all denizens of the otherworld were pink and glittery) if it was consumed as a soup or in pancake form on the feast day of St. John the Baptist, meaning around the summer solstice.

Stinging Nettle Pancakes

I have been a passionate cook since childhood, and this is a recipe I can't give exact measurements on. I always eyeball nettle pancakes.

You will need:

One to two eggs

Flour

Milk

Dried or freshly chopped stinging nettle leaves

Salt, pepper, and spices (according to taste)

Oil for frying

Take a big bowl and add the egg, a handful of stinging nettle leaves and a little milk. Mix the ingredients well with a whisk. Take a sieve and add a little flour. Continue, sifting in the flour little by little to avoid clumps. Perhaps add a little more milk until you have reached the desired amount. The batter is perfect when it is a thick liquid without being too firm—a little like the consistency of toothpaste. Add spices according to taste and add more leaves if it is not green enough for you.

Heat a pan over medium heat, add a little oil and fry the pancakes until they are golden brown on each side.

The first one is for the proverbial dog, meaning the first flapjack often does not turn out very well, but after the second things begin to flow nicely. If you prefer your pancakes extra fluffy, separate the egg and only stir the egg yolk into the batter. Keep the egg white aside until you are done with the batter, then beat until stiff and carefully fold it in just before you begin to make the pancakes.

You can generally use stinging nettle as an herb in the kitchen. They don't necessarily have a strong taste, but add a healing effect to your dishes.

Stinging Nettle Water for Hair Loss

It is best to freshly prepare the stinging nettle water. Mixtures with alcohol tend to additionally irritate the scalp and oil extracts have to be rinsed out, which is stressful on the skin as well.

Pour one to two liters of boiling water over one to two handfuls of dried nettles and let steep until the liquid has cooled to lukewarm. Next, strain out the nettles and use the liquid as the final treatment after shampooing your hair. Gently massage it into your scalp and do not rinse it out.

Do this once a week and drink stinging nettle tea on a semi-regular basis and your hair will recover quickly.

St. John's Wort
(Hypericum perforatum)

There is little left to be added to the discussion of St. John's wort. Only the terminology has changed; what used to be considered an herb that could ward off demons is described as an antidepressant today.

St. John's wort is a plant of light through and through. It is so full of light that it makes people more sensitive to light as well. This means you should avoid sunbathing when you are consuming St. John's wort.

If you are taking birth control pills, you should not take St. John's wort; even other medications could have unwanted interactions with this herb. You should consult your doctor or pharmacist in those cases. Even though I generally make the case for a relaxed management of herbs, they should be taken seriously. Even plants can interact with medications.

St. John's wort takes one to two weeks for its effects to unfold and thus is one of those plants whose effects build up step by step.

In the old days it was used to cure infections alongside its mood-lifting qualities. This encompassed the whole body: the mouth, the intestinal tract, the kidneys, and the bladder. For a scratchy throat or a developing cough, gargle with St. John's wort. It acts as a disinfectant and wards off infection.

St. John's wort was further considered a natural potency remedy for both sexes. It was used against manipulative love spells, for which it can be useful to this day. Its red extract was seen as a symbol for blood and people connected it to Mary, Joseph, and John (whose name it bears).

Breaking Magic Spells and Streaks of Bad Luck with St. John's Wort

When you have the feeling that everything around you is bewitched, St. John's wort is among the helpers that effectively drive away this hazy veil.

People often make the mistake of looking to the outside when they believe someone bewitched them. The rule is: even when someone has bewitched you, the important thing is how *you* deal with it. After all, you can option to refuse acceptance, and return to sender. The only thing that matters is how you deal with it in your head. No one can bewitch a person who has closed all doors to it. When in doubt, remember it is fear that opens this door.

But a string of bad luck can make life difficult. Smudge your home with St. John's wort in this case and thoroughly mop through it after adding St. John's wort to the mop bucket. Sprinkle a little St. John's wort tea on the window sills and all thresholds, perhaps even out by the garden gate. Afterward take a candle made of beeswax, write the names of all members of your household (including pets if they are like family members) on it, and apply St. John's wort oil to it. To make the oil, leave the herb in a carrier oil for two weeks; or just buy some ready-made, which you can find in the pharmacy or health food store in capsule form.

Valerian ⊘

(Valeriana officinalis)

Travelling herb peddlers used to tell their alpine customers, "The day ends and the day begins with a pinch of valerian." I would not recommend it for daily use, however. It is rather a plant for times of crisis and can also be used as a little relaxation treatment. Be careful not to use it over long periods of time. In the case of continuous tension, you will simply have to change something about your life. No plant can keep absorbing that. Valerian works against anxiety and sleep troubles. It is one of the most powerful nerve herbs and is ideal for trying situations. It can also lend support in cases of headaches, menstrual pain, and migraines.

Due to its relaxing effect, valerian was also valued as an aphrodisiac (only those who are truly relaxed can have a clear head for love). Valerian can serve as a soft brake that reduces the pressure of the daily routine and returns us again to our relaxed normal state. In magic valerian is considered a plant against evil. Its strong aroma dispels anything that is less than good-natured.

Migraine Combo

When it comes to migraines, valerian and lavender work extremely well together. Take valerian tablets in accordance with the package directions or make a cup of valerian tea, meaning one teaspoon valerian root per cup; let it steep for ten minutes, then drink in small sips, preferably warm. After taking the tea or pills, drip lavender oil on a handkerchief and find a quiet, dark place. Breathe in the lavender smell as long as it is agreeable.

Should you be nauseous from the migraine, you can add a drop of mint oil.

This combination will not magically make the migraine disappear, but it will certainly shorten it and reduce the severity of the attack.

Techniques for Using Herbs

As promised, here are general tips for the preparation and use of plants.

Tea

Measure a heaping teaspoonful of the herb per cup of boiling water and let the tea steep for seven to ten minutes. If you are working with an aromatic plant whose essential oils are central to its effect (lavender, rosemary, thyme, and linden blossoms, for example), you should cover the cup while steeping. You don't have to cover the tea if you are working with non-aromatic plants—horsetail, oak bark, or calendula, for example.

Salve and Oil with Dried Herbs

Add one ounce of dried herbs to about one cup of salve base (Vaseline, Shea butter, clarified butter, or lard, for example) or one cup of oil (almond oil, coconut oil, or similar). Carefully heat them in a bain-marie and strain them out and fill containers afterward. As soon as the salve cools down, you can add a little essential oil if you wish to mildly scent it. Store in a cool, dark place.

Oil Infused with Fresh Herbs

Add fresh herbs to sufficient oil (about two ounces of herbs to one cup oil, or eyeball it) in a vessel with a wide neck. Do not cover it with a lid, but with a clean cloth or a sieve; the mixture must be able to breathe so that all the moisture from the herbs evaporates, otherwise it may begin to mold. The herbs should remain in the oil for about two weeks, during which time the vessel must remain warm. If whitish streaks appear, it must be heated briefly (heater, hairdryer) until the oil is clear once more. These infused oils are very aromatic and can easily be used in the kitchen, made from basil and similar herbs.

Essential Oils

As mentioned before, essential oils should be carefully chosen; they are highly concentrated substances that are not found in this form in nature, but are dispersed throughout the entire plant. Most oils are not dangerous when used with a scent lamp, but as a rule you should read about them, preferably from multiple sources, before you utilize your essence of choice.

Those who do not want to use a scent lamp or essential oil burner because of the open flame or for other reasons often use a diffuser instead, with varying results. Try using cork instead, such as cork coasters or thin cork tiles from a craft supply store. You can dab them with oils and hang them like an air freshener. Cork releases the scent wonderfully and is not very expensive. Homemade cork hangers like this can also be sprinkled with cedar or lavender oil and used against moths in the closet.

Bath

For an herbal bath, add two handfuls of the dried herb to a big pot of boiling water (about three quarts). Next, take it off the stove and let the whole thing steep (with a tight-fitting lid) for about fifteen minutes before you add it to the bath water. Don't use any other additives. Bathe in it for about twenty minutes. The water level should not be higher than the heart.

If you want to use tougher ingredients (roots, horsetail, oak bark) boil them for ten minutes, then take the pot off the stove and only then add (if you wish) the more tender plant parts to let it steep with the rest. You have to be sensible when you combine these things: the comparatively tender basil or scented blossoms would lose their aromatic components after ten minutes in boiling water while the harder horsetail needs to be boiled for quite a while so that its active ingredients can be properly released.

Incense

Add the dried plant parts of choice to an incense coal or a teapot warmer and let them burn. You don't always need the full equipment. You can also hold a piece of aluminum foil over the flame from a candle. Start with no more than the amount that fits on the tip of a knife. You can always add more later. Besides its overall cleansing effect, incense can symbolically smoke out the spirit of a sickness and thus dispel it.

Amulet

Old books about herbs naturally reason that one herb is best worn on the arm, another should be tied to the leg, while a third should be worn on the chest. This is based on the old knowledge of herbs; they are not only ingredients to be consumed in order to feel something, but plant beings as well who transmit effects through their own personality.

Carry them on you in a little sachet or wrapped in a cloth, for example, in your bra, pants pocket, or handbag. Basically, the closer you carry it on your body, the better. Wear it directly on your skin if you can.

If you feel a special connection to an herb you can also stick it to your body under a band-aid during your normal everyday routine if it has to be especially discreet and work clothes don't allow for enough flexibility. In the old days roots and such were often enclosed in silver or gold and worn as pendants. If that is not a possibility, simply carry them as close to you as possible. Just do what is practical for you; it is hard to imagine that a distance of a few centimeters would present an insurmountable obstacle for the sympathetic spirit of a plant.

Spiritual Possibilities

We can work with plants on a purely spiritual level by meditating in front of a plant or its picture, for example. You will not always receive an instant response. Sometimes these messages arrive later in a dream or in the form of meaningful coincidences. This should not be considered in a linear, cause-and-effect way, for example thinking that something should happen any minute. Instead, look at it this way: when you sit down and internally make contact with a plant's energy, you open a door. That does not necessarily mean someone is going to walk through it instantly, although this can occasionally happen. Everything takes time. When working with multiple plants, you will notice that some of them are immediately tangible while others are silent for a long time. Be patient with yourself and the plant spirits.

In our everyday routines, most of us feel that everything has to happen quickly and be perfect. Mistakes are not acceptable and delays are even worse. We have to shed this mentality when we begin to work on the internal plane. It is not always easy to change our thinking in this way. Don't be discouraged if this does not work immediately. Practice in playful earnest, as I like to call it, earnest because you are serious about it, and playful because this attitude opens the path, clears it of obstacles, and shuts down those expectations of perfection that we often carry with us from childhood on.

Another way to get closer to plants is to paint or draw them. In my experience this is one of the deepest reaching possibilities because the hands translate the energy of the plant in a completely different way than we do it with the head. You don't have to have any special drawing "ability" to do this. Forget about talent or skill for a minute and assume that you are completely free in your artistic expression. In reality we are all free to do this. We simply don't have the guts to laugh about the ridiculous evaluation of others in terms of what is supposedly "beautiful" or "ugly" and simply do what is fun for us.

You think you draw like a six-year-old? What's the problem? Have you seen the beautiful pictures children can draw? The painter Wassily Kandinsky spent years of his life studying the drawings of children. Franz Marc exhibited his paintings next to those of children and Paul Klee found inspiration in the drawings of his small son. August Macke asked if children are possibly more creative "in drawing directly from the secret of their sensations?" [48] And with that he has hit exactly upon

48. August Macke, "Masks." Art Theory. http://theoria.art-zoo.com/masks-august-macke/Accessed Oct. 25, 2017. Originally published in Der Blaue Reiter Almanach (The Blue Rider Almanac) in 1912.

the subject we are all trying to reach: creating out of the secret of perception, making the invisible visible, giving it a language not made of words but of colors and forms instead.

You can portray a plant's energy in an abstract way with color gradients; you can glue a collage together or scribble it with a pencil. If you are shy, get yourself some finger paints and packing paper and work with that. Think about how happy children are when they do this, and get started.

You don't have to show your pictures to anyone. No one has the right to judge them. If you don't consider your picture to be a success, keep it for a few more days. Don't throw it out right away. This is not about supposed beauty or images that show every exact detail or proportion. It is about an energetic image of the plant. This is completely different. Think about the drawings of shamans in tribal art and cave paintings. Only use these as an initial inspiration, though. Don't copy things, but do your own thing. Whatever comes, it is okay. If you don't think it turned out okay at first glance, wait a little bit until your viewpoint has softened and you will be able to tell that it is expressing something after all. The art is in the ability to let the picture remain as it is.

This also means not analyzing it to death. If you realize something from the picture, excellent. If you find out things about the plant that you were unaware of before, wonderful. However, don't pick it apart: this isn't psychoanalysis, but shamanic drawing. It is not about your state of mind, but about finding another expression for the things that you see in a plant by means of the body and the hands. If you have a problem allowing yourself to do it initially, start with tackling it for only five minutes at a time. This is a little trick that turns off the critical voice in your head. After five minutes people are often deep in the creative flow or at the very least curious enough to continue trying.

Magical Stones and More

We can draw from a wide variety of stones today, but even our ancestors had their favorites among stones when it came to healing work and protection. If we want to take a closer look at stones, we have to take a few steps back into their time. Back then you couldn't walk into a store or shop online in order to simply buy your stone of choice. Stones were something special, and simply by being special it was easier to use them for healing work. Not everything was available all the time and that's why people recognized the value of it. Often magical stones (typically contained in jewelry) were inherited over generations, which gave them additional power. What helped my grandmother will help me too—these opened completely different doors than anonymous stones purchased in a store. Many magical instructions from the old days emphasize that one should use a family heirloom if possible.

This is more difficult for us today than it was for our ancestors. We can attain so many things with ease if we have the necessary funds, but that is precisely what makes it difficult to find items to use in magic: things that are readily available are not *special*.

I already mentioned how important mental images are in healing work; both head and heart want to be enchanted. This is when the doors to self-healing powers open. In the old days, peddlers who told their customers the most amazing stories about the origin of the stones they sold did people a favor. People (who certainly didn't believe everything but were well entertained) began to dream and allowed the stone into their heart. Today, we would say, "What a charlatan! The stones are certainly not from the treasure of an Indian princess. The stones origi-nated in a mine in Brazil. I won't be fooled."

We have to admit that we still let ourselves be fooled and want to dream. One example is the highly praised Himalayan salt that is often or-dinary rock salt that comes from Poland, yet it costs twenty times what normal salt costs. Some will object that it works well for them and that is exactly what I am talking about: if you value something, it has a ret-roactive effect. Do we enchant ourselves by believing in something, de-veloping cozy, positive images and emotions to go along with it and thus ascribe extra value to it? Yes, and that is a good thing. How we activate self-healing powers is irrelevant as long as it works and does no harm.

Many of the stones used by our ancestors are fossils. We find those as far back as the earliest graves in history, as well as over and over again in ancient jewelry finds. Therefore, if we pick up work with fossils today we step into an ancient stream of knowledge.

Of course, the following is true here as well: we will feel a sense of chemistry with some things and not others. This is no different than it is with plants and other healing methods. Traditions that have been handed down are one thing, but they only represent a fraction of the possibilities, and the ultimate importance is where the spark travels and the feeling that something works. This is where the energy begins to flow.

Fossilized Ammonite

(also: Snake Egg, Dragon Stone, Wheel of the Gods)

Fossilized ammonites were popular protection stones due to their spi-ral and snake symbolism. Big ammonites can be found on house walls in rural France and England, either constructed into the wall or in the form of paintings on walls that depict the symbolism. Magical ammo-nite amulets were used whenever something needed special protection or was supposed to go well. They were (and still are) an excellent means of support in terms of regaining health.

Even today they are said to help with unfulfilled wishes of childbirth and are considered a kind of fossilized aphrodisiac. As such, you can carry a small specimen with you as an amulet, fasten it to your bed, or place it on your nightstand. Those who need a more discreet solution can also lay an ammonite under their mattress.

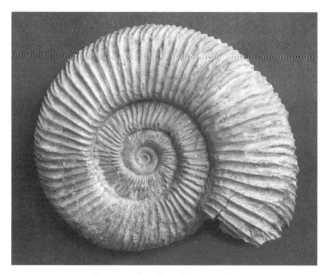

Figure 1: fossilized ammonite

They were used as oracle stones in ancient Egypt. Especially pyritized ammonites (those bonded to pyrite), which are known as "golden snails" in Germany today, were considered stones of priests. In many cultures they have a connection to meditation and the path to enlightenment. But even in everyday life they hold a strong "lightbulb moment" energy. Ammonites can be wonderful support during uncertainties of any kind, when you do not know your path or want to examine underlying causes.

Belemnites

(Bullet Stones, Devil's Fingers, St. Peter's Fingers,
Thunderbolt, Ghostly Candles;
additionally in German folk vernacular:
Lynx Stone, Fright Stone)

Belemnite guard fossils are the fossilized ancestors of today's squid. In the old folk traditions of Germany, they were most often called Thunderbolts, and carried a special significance against bewitching and for protection against illness in general. In Northern Germany, especially, they were worn as amulets well into the present time. The stones are considered helpful against fright as the cause for an illness (which today we might call a psychosomatic trigger). Thunderbolts are classic stones for spells. It is documented that in the former regions of Prussia, Pomerania, and Saxony, physicians used them to cure bladder stones by incantation.[49]

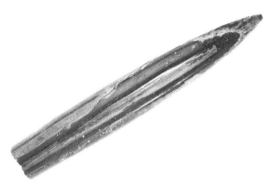

Figure 2: belemnite fossil

Their use is not limited to that, however. They were also used to brush warts in folk medicine; three times in the form of a cross, preferably on a Thursday or Sunday.

Belemnites can be used to brush away multiple ailments and then to seal the spot with three cross-like motions. The stone thus supports the healing power of the hand.

As always, the rule here is that simply copying what our ancestors used to do does not necessarily help us reach the goal. We should consider the old traditions as an inspiration, but never forget to use our common sense and our intuition here and now in order to apply old knowledge in contemporary ways.

---

49. Schmidt, 79

Jet

(Black Amber)

Jet is also of fossilized origin. It was sometimes called "black amber" because it feels similar to amber. In actuality the two are not far removed from one another. Jet is fossilized plant material, a form of coal formed from pressurized decomposition of wood, while amber is fossilized tree resin.

In German-speaking regions it is known as widow's stone. It has been documented as the favored jewelry during times of grief ever since the Middle Ages. Jet is not only protective for those in mourning, but for little children as well. Basically, jet is a stone which helps anyone who is more vulnerable than others, whether this is due to their young age, a particular sensitivity, or a personal situation. It is like a filter that repels negativity. It is also used against the evil eye, envy, and streaks of bad luck, and protects what is near and dear to us. This refers not only to health, but also to personal belongings and our dearest relatives.

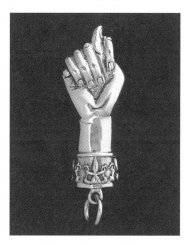

Figure 3: mano figa

In regions where Romance languages are spoken, we see the *mano figa azabache*, meaning a Figa hand (a hand with the thumb tucked between the index and middle fingers) made from jet. This is often decorated with a bead made from luck-bringing coral, other red beads or gems, or a red cord, and it protects against all evil. It particularly protects against the *mal de ojo*, the evil eye. Sometimes the hand can be found carved from coral.

Germanic people are said to have picked up the hand as a good luck symbol. It is called the "fig of envy" in German. It is easy to see that the hand gesture symbolically hints at intercourse, and offensive and sexual allusions have always been considered apotropaic in folk traditions, meaning they ward off spells or evil. In Slavic and Russian regions, this gesture simply means "no" and as such is an entirely neutral defense.

Hematite

Hematite is also known as "blood stone" in Germany (not to be confused with bloodstone), since the stone's grinding water takes on a red tint when the stone is polished. It was used to cure bleeding magically and was generally considered a stone that strengthens vitality, because what is good for the blood is also good for the whole human being.

Snake Stones and Snake Eggs

(Fossilized Sea Urchins, Echinoids; also, in German folk vernacular:
Victory Stone, Thunder Stone, Stone of the Gods, Soul Stone,
Toad Stone, Sea Apple, Druid's Stone)

Snake Eggs, or Snake Stones, are fossilized sea urchins with five-pointed star designs or bumps. They can look very different; some are fairly flat, almost like sand dollars, while others are pointed or bumpy. They have been found as grave goods since the Bronze Age. They are therefore also soul stones, which are connected to the power of the ancestors.

Snake stones containing star shapes were very popular until the eighteenth century as an all-around amulet and were sometimes worn as jewelry, partially encased in silver or gold. The star-shaped pattern is reminiscent of a pentagram, which was considered a reliable remedy against nightmares and the so-called *druden* (pressure ghosts that torment people in the night so that they wake up exhausted the next morning). This is still true in many rural regions today. Snake stones are said to protect against evil spirits, which used to include demons of illnesses.

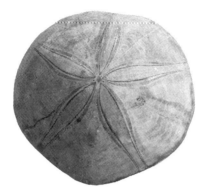

Figure 4: echinoid fossil

In modern times there are other stones (ammonite or serpentine, for example) that are referred to as snake stone. Do not be confused by this. It is apparent when reading the old texts that the term "snake stone" in German was almost interchangeably used with "power stone" or "magic stone," regardless of the actual stone in question. We can find a possible explanation for the popularity of "snake" stones in the shamanic worldview. When demons of illness are considered "worms" in the body, a snake stone can speak to them, move them, and help lead them out of the body.

Fossilized sea urchins which show small bumps in a radiating pattern (known in German as Snake Eggs or Druid's Stone, in English folk vernacular as chalk eggs, sugar loaves, or fairy loaves) were the magic stones of the Druids according to Pliny the Elder. Among the general population they were known as stones of protection.

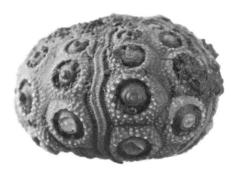

Figure 5: fossilized sea urchin, bumpy variety

"Protection" seems a little vague to us today. Which areas of application? How exactly? Where exactly? I want it exactly, down to the gram, to the spell, to the gesture!

With an anxious, demanding attitude like that you will not get to the bottom of secrets like these. They want to be sensed; they need to be found by a loving search party that is willing to experiment, extend their antennae and trust in their gut feeling. A personal connection to the item that is being used is necessary, too. It does not work to simply buy everything quickly to file it away in a mental type case to be sorted by its associated effect. This is no way to discover the powers of stones and fossils.

Let it in, follow your feelings, listen to your instincts. Is the chemistry right? Is anything getting across at all? Not every stone is made for everybody. Even a super stone can be silent for some people, while a simple stone on the side of the road can be brimming with power and energy. Do not think about price, rarity, touted effects or the like. Don't let that cloud your view of the actual strength of the stone. Also consider that each individual stone is different; we may warm up toward a certain specimen of a type of rock or mineral, while others leave us cold. Even if you don't happen to feel a connection to a stone, maybe someone in your inner circle will connect with it.

Returning stones back to nature is also possible if the chemistry is not right; many a stone will thank you for its freedom more than if you cling forcefully to it. Especially since stones are not necessarily gone once you return them to nature. I used to have a stone which I could sense insisted on being in a river. This wasn't easy for me because I liked it a lot, but I eventually granted its wish. I can feel its distinctive energy to this day as if a good spirit were stopping by. If I had known that ahead of time, it wouldn't have been so hard for me to let it go.

Tongue stones

(Fossilized shark teeth; in German folk vernacular,
Colubrid Stones, Colubrid Tongues)

Tongue stones are nothing more than fossilized shark teeth. They can often be found in surfer jewelry. They ward off the evil eye and enemies (even an illness can be an enemy in this sense). In the old days they were considered amulets against speech problems—*nomen est omen*—they were supposed to loosen the tongue. Today we know that they are fossilized teeth, not tongues, but that does not take away anything from their effect. The shark is truly not a bad ally when it comes to warding off negative energy.

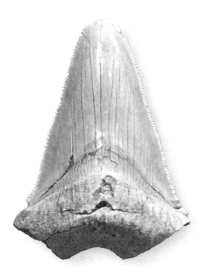

Figure 6: tongue stone
aka shark tooth fossil

The Magical Duo: Turquoise and Coral

Turquoise and coral play an important role in magical jewelry. This color pattern is not only found in Europe, but also in Nepal, Tibet, with Native Americans, and with the Romany and other Travelers. Turquoise and coral are blue and red stones that are worn together and have an especially protecting and healing effect. Jewelry in the old folk traditions sometimes used azurite or azurmalachite as an alternative for turquoise, or people worked with blue and red glass beads.

These two stones symbolize the polarity of life. Blue is the feminine color (consider the blue starry cloak of the virgin Mary) and red is the masculine color (many painters picked up this knowledge and expressed it in the red sash over Jesus's white robes). This is echoed in the magical tradition, with red as the color of Mars and blue as the color of Venus (next to green ... it depends on the specific tradition). Romany and Travelers also consider blue to be the color of the woman and red the color of the man while purple, as their union, is used especially for calming and relaxation.

Purple balances out the opposites. It is not only a spiritual, but also an extremely harmonizing color. Everything in moderation, however! If you surrounded yourself only with purple all that harmony would render you limp and lazy. We need the stimulus and the ups and downs of change in life in order to be truly alive.

Turquoise stands for water, the sky, and the air, while coral represents blood, fire, and light. In both past and present turquoise and coral were used as protecting, healing stones. They work like a yin and yang in color, helping to restore you to your natural balance. Both stones have been considered reliable detectors of when something is not right with the person wearing them. In this case the stones become noticeably pale or the opposite, noticeably dark, or they may lose their luster or break. Those who work with stones will have had experiences like this; after all, stones are anything but inanimate objects of nature.

One can also meditate wonderfully on the polarity of life with both stones. Ideally, use them together, not individually. Even if we sometimes have the wish to be especially dynamic and strong (red) or soft and balanced (blue), ultimately, we always need both parts in order to be whole. These two stones can be used as jewelry or carried in pant pockets, and can lend support during any chronic or unclear illness, as well as for overall loss of energy and nervous problems. The stones should be worn close to the body if possible. In traditional jewelry from India or in Native American traditions, both stones are often set together.

Fossilized Coral

(also in German: Star Stone, Spider Stone, Jinx Stone)

Fossilized coral used to be sold in polished form, particularly when carved in a heart shape, which was considered effective help against jinxes and was used as a counter-spell to avert all evil. Of course, you can use them in any other shape as well.

Because of their texture they were also known as star stone or spider stone. They were used to stanch bleeding, among other things. Nowadays we go to the doctor for that, but you can still test fossilized coral's good reputation for helping resolve skin rashes and problems of any kind today. As a rule, these stones not only bring order and structure to the tissue, but to thoughts as well.

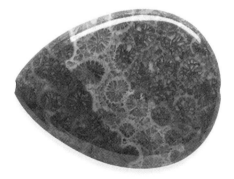

Figure 7: fossilized coral

Hag Stones/Holey Stones

(witch stones, adder stones;
also in German folk vernacular: chicken gods)

Chicken gods are stones with a natural hole in the middle. They are primarily found by the seaside. These are old luck talismans and avert harm of any kind. An old man living on the island of Rügen told me that they contain an old healing magic. If you look through the hole at the sun it is supposed to free you of illness and soothe any existing discomforts.

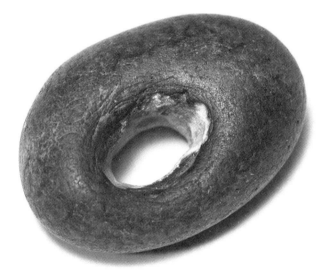

Figure 8: holey stone

Chalk

Chalk used to be more than just a white stone. It used to be stirred into salves (just like healing earth, which is made up of loess) that were supposed to heal the most diverse list of ailments. The healing power of the minerals played a decisive role in all this. Chalk was also used in more magical healing cures in order to draw a boundary around and protect the sick person. People also drew signs and symbols with it to bless house and farm. In Germany, it is still a familiar tradition in many regions for groups of people called "star singers" to go from house to house on Epiphany (January 6), writing blessings onto houses with chalk.

Red Stones

Red stones have had a special significance in healing magic for a long time. Red is the color of life and according to old beliefs it fends off any powers of a hostile nature. A fair number of red things were utilized, from valuable ruby to garnet, coral, carnelian, and even red glass beads. Red string, necklaces, cloth, stitching and ribbons were used against illnesses and to prevent ailments.

We can still do this today wonderfully. You can tie a little red ribbon or string to yourself, wear jewelry with red stones or (glass) beads, or purposely choose red pieces of clothing. Italians wear red underwear on New Year's Eve because it brings them good luck for the New Year.

If red is not necessarily your color, you can also discreetly hide it under your clothing. No one will notice a small band around an ankle. You just have to be a little creative. Especially at times when you feel weak—not completely fit, but not really sick—red can help you get back on your feet. It is also a wonderful color for the little ones. It protects them.

Bricks/Masonry of Special Buildings

When we speak of red bricks we basically return to the symbolism of red stones in general; however, this time the focus is on abraded dust, or brick powder. Due to the high iron content (which causes the redness during the firing process) it is possible that the invigorating effect is true, even though I would not recommend simply pulverizing bricks and consuming the product today. This dust was sometimes worked into salves and was considered an all-around healing remedy against pretty much any ailment.

Powder from church stonework was also believed to have healing powers, especially when it was acquired in the vicinity of the altar. Unexplainable grooves that confirm this custom exist in many old churches to this day. The time around Easter, Christmas, and the twelve days of

Christmas were considered to bring the most luck for this endeavor. Some traditions point even further back in history; in Southern Europe people used to fire special clay figures from which powder was scraped off that would then be mixed into food or salves for healing purposes.[50]

Metal

My grandmother used the biggest kitchen knife she could find whenever one of us kids managed to get a bump on the head. I can remember how scared I was the first time, because I thought she wanted to cut the bump off. The whole thing was not so bad after all and I didn't get even the slightest bruise. The knife was simply pressed to the aching spot and held there for a little while. The explanation was that the knife cools the spot, but other cool things would have been just as effective. After reading about many magical techniques involving a knife to banish illnesses, I think this is an older technique that became rationalized over time ("it is cooling").

Later on, I read about a tradition collected by the researcher of Romany customs, Heinrich von Wlislocki,[51] that describes the exact same approach and is even connected to a spell. Even then people used to press a knife to the aching area and recite the following spell three, seven, or nine times (depending on the severity of the bump).

Soften, soften, soften up,
And disappear at once!
You shall go to the Earth,
Never to be seen again!

---

50. Schmidt, 81
51. Von Wlislocki, *Magic Formulas and Incantations…*, 58.

Knife, knife, draw it out,
Hand it over to the earth![52]

Afterward the knife was plunged into the Earth three, seven, or nine times and pulled out again. With or without the spell, the use of the knife was effective every time; this is perhaps due to the impression of a large kitchen knife, which tends to draw every child's attention to it immediately. I still like to lay a knife on spots that I've bumped to this day. It simply works too well, and I don't care if it is imprinted from early childhood, superstition, or verified in some way. The deciding factor is that it is effective. If you try it yourself you will feel a slightly uncomfortable feeling at first, changing into a somehow electrical feeling (it's difficult to put into words), as if the pain were wandering into the knife.

Similarly, the application of an axe also works. It was used as a type of threat to the sickness spirit. A (fairly dull) axe is placed flat on the affected area and kept there for a few minutes. In some areas the custom was to place the blade of a knife flat on the back of one's neck in order to stop a nosebleed. This is often still done with a set of keys today.

Keys also played a role in the old healing traditions; during calf cramps one was supposed to stroke the cramping area with a key. The older the key, the better it was. Several "bone breakers" in Eastern Friesland (the traditional name for bone setters in that area) still use this method with horses that require treatment. Originally this widely spread method was also used on humans. Another custom said that to banish an illness, a sick person should hammer three nails (into a wood block, for example) with all their might.

---

52. Charles Godfrey Leland gives this translation of the charm in his *Gypsy Sorcery and Fortunetelling*:
"Be thou, be thou, be thou weak (i.e., soft)
And very soon perish!
Go thou into the earth,
May I see thee never more
Bring knives, knives,
Give (i.e., put) into the earth."

Back when people used to use fire strikers or fire steels to start a fire, they were used for inflammations, in keeping with the belief that an item that has a specific effect (in this case to start a fire) also has the ability to take it away (here: the fire of the inflammation). Fire strikers seem to have been a very popular remedy. They were also placed on tumors, broken bones, and headaches. It is obvious that we should reasonably go to the doctor in cases like this today, although the additional application can't hurt. Fire strikers can be purchased at Renaissance fairs and via the internet.

A Few Tips
for Getting Started

The principle for healing work of any kind is this: as much as necessary, but as little as possible. You should also stick to this rule when it comes to magical healing work, since body, mind, and soul should be nudged to do their own job rather than weakened, which can result if we ease their burden too much. "Use it or lose it." This work is not about spinning a soft healing cocoon around ourselves, but about getting fit again, so we can stand up to our daily lives as well as possible.

Sometimes relief is the first and most important goal. Not everything can be healed completely, even if the trend of believing everything is possible spins fine yarns in this regard. A friend who is a physical therapist developed a system for her work which you can use or adapt as needed. Since many patients come to her with the expectation "now fix me right away" and like to announce their displeasure when decades of stress or strain fail to disappear in a single session, she asks patients to estimate how they are feeling before the session on a scale from one (really bad) to ten (excellent). She asks them after the session which point of the scale they see themselves at now. This shows much more realistic results.

Don't try to "collect" every available method, but rather concentrate on that which truly moves you forward, and polish it over time. We often subscribe to the erroneous belief that everyone has to know as many methods as possible. The old healers viewed that very differently.

They had their pet subjects, but there were also areas in which they deferred to other people because it was simply not their area of expertise. They knew their limitations and knew that it is normal to have some limitations.

Having such an attitude does not mean that you are a bad healer. If you are extremely good at something and are well versed in it, it is a thousand times more valuable than knowing a little bit about twenty techniques. Psychology also comes into play here. When you help someone and are sure of what you are doing, the other person will perceive you very differently than if you are unsure of yourself. This goes for yourself as well, since you can't fool yourself.

Under no circumstances should you start healing work with any sense of vanity, overestimating your capabilities because you want to look good. Stay courageous, but humble. Don't let others put you on a pedestal or put pressure on you even if you have a sure hand for some things. This is important because we tend to put pressure on ourselves to the tune of: "It has always worked. Hopefully it will work this time as well."

Over time you will develop an intuition about how to proceed. Think about who and what you want to include, and respect your personal preferences. You don't have to be instantly good at everything. Not everyone likes plants, stones, or wants to lay hands on people. Find your own way. As a little help for starting out, I made up a little list of questions for you.

- Which spiritual power/presence do I want to bring aboard? Do I want to skip this for now?
- Are there certain stones I would like to use?
- Should plants be involved and if yes, what kind and in which form?
- Do I wish to use a spell?
- Do I want to lay my hands on someone or work with direct contact (blowing, stroking, brushing, etc.)?
- Would I rather work magically with symbols and candles?

- Will nature be involved, for example, by leaving symbols of the illness at rivers, trees, or special places, or do I want to magically pass on ailments?
- Do I want to incorporate the days of the week and the phase of the moon?

If you are unsure, stick to the formula "less is more." It does not help to pile on multiple methods. It is important simply that you truly feel something and can tell by the results that you are making progress. This is your path. Don't expect it to happen instantly. A lot of people are too impatient. I will exaggerate a bit to make my point: they want to read a book and be a good healer afterward. It's a nice idea, but how is that supposed to happen? You can't gain experience from a book. You can only gain it by *doing*. This requires time, patience, and commitment.

Let's assume you are working with a spell and experience success with it. You have gained important experience, namely the fact that it can work. You are now in a different position than before when a book promised you that it works, but you still had your doubts that it was possible. So you continue your path and try out other spells. Over time you will find out which areas suit you and which questions seem to lead you nowhere. You will learn the talents and gifts that you were given, and surprises are sure to find you along the way. You walk your path in life, not in a book. Your inner spirit will awaken and start to pull you toward experiences and information that will be helpful for your further development. Sometimes they can even come in the proverbial form of problems that are opportunities in disguise.

The nuts you will need to crack in order to move ahead are often very hard.

Don't throw in the towel too soon, but allow yourself to be present and patient. A lot of people get nervous when something doesn't happen for them right away and they immediately give up on the whole subject. Instead, stay vigilant and see if you can't learn something from the whole experience. Such stumbling blocks are often like tests and, as a thank you, a door opens afterward. Sometimes the timing isn't right, but that does not mean you should then abandon the whole matter. If a subject is truly important for your path, if it is fate of some kind, it will find you again. You may not have a use for it immediately. It may take weeks, months, or years. Subjects like this are like seeds that slumber in the earth; when the conditions are right they will one day sprout and grow. You won't lose anything. What is truly important rests within you already. It cannot be forgotten or overlooked because it will come to life on its own when the time is right.

If you prefer to work for others, respect their preferences and life circumstances. A lot depends on the familiarity you have with each other. As an example, I once heard of a man who thought it was horrible to have hands laid on him. It felt uncomfortable to him, but he did not say anything because he thought this was the way it had to be. Issues like this can only happen when people do not clearly discuss their expectations and the course of the treatment ahead of time. Apparently even during the man's session there was no room to discuss this. Open communication is vitally important in healing sessions. What are your expectations? What is the procedure? Are both sides okay with it?

Distance Healing

Those who think the subject of distance healing is a modern development are wrong. Distance healing was common in the old days as well. When a patient was too sick to make the trip to see the healer, friends and relatives went instead to ask for help for the sick person. They often brought a few hairs, nail clippings or similar things with them, so that the healing work could be specifically tailored to the patient. Nowadays people primarily use photos.

Of course, all this carried with it the sensitive question of what to do if people request help on behalf of a sick person who is unaware of the request? What to do with a worried mother, for instance, who would like her daughter to be worked on even though the daughter is against alternative healing methods and would consider her mother's endeavor laughable hocus pocus? Or what to do when someone cannot communicate due to health reasons and cannot answer questions?

There are several different approaches to this. Some healers flat out refuse to work with cases like these while others have no problems with it and are happy to help.

In the old days people were of the opinion that if the illness is bad, it needs to go. Today we tend to start ruminating on whether or not the illness could possibly serve as a warning to the patient and may help them change his or her behavior (I am not speaking of "karma" or what most people understand it to be, or of guilt, but of instances where people may have an epiphany). If we begin working with it and thus shorten the illness, we may deprive the individual of an important process of realization.

As I wrote about in my book *Magie Leben* (*Living Magic),* I do believe that we can work for this patient; however, it should be without specifying which path the energy should take. Figuratively speaking, this is like creating an energy depot for someone while letting the subconscious of the person decide if and how it will accept the energy.

You will need a connection to the affected person in order to do distance healing. It can be a name or a birthday, but also hair, nails, worn clothing, writing samples and many other things are imaginable. A photo is ideal, of course. One depicting the whole body is best. The affected area should be on the photo. If someone has back problems, for example, it is recommended that the photo shows the person from behind. The person can be dressed in normal clothing, of course. What's important is simply that the person can be seen from head to toe and that the affected area is in the picture.

I am ending this book with an old book theft blessing I found by accident during my research. Finding thieves and preventing theft was actually an additional job for many healers in the old days, as surprising as this may sound today (but not so surprising if we see that shamans do exactly the same things even in modern times).

Theft was a widespread problem in the old days; doors with secure locks did not exist back then. The so-called theft blessing was supposed to prevent such pilfering. Healers were often active in warding off thieves as well. Precious as books were in these days, they had to be especially secured.

> This book is loved beyond belief
> He who steals it is a thief.
> Be he a lord or be he serf,
> The gallows are what he deserves.
> Should he come upon a house,
> He will thence be chased right out.
> Should he find a ditch as haven,
> He will be eaten by ravens.
> Should he come upon a stone,
> He will break his neck and bone.

Appendix:
Sympathy, Antipathy,
and Magnetism

Sympathy used to be and still is simply another word for magic in many rural areas. This is where terms like sympathy and black sympathy originated (we would call it white or black magic today).

The belief in sympathy makes the basic assumption that everything has a soul or a kind of energy vibration. Therefore, some things are sympathetic or familiar to each other based on their similar vibration. A warming plant like ginger, for example, has an excellent effect on feverish colds because it fights fire with fire.

Antipathy is considered healing through opposites in folk medicine. In this case cooling plants like mint and eucalyptus are used to combat colds accompanied by fever. The neutralization that occurs when two separate influences act on each other and create equilibrium is key here. Hot and cold create lukewarm.

Folk magic utilized both principles equally. No strict blanket formulas exist about which variation to use when. In general, the healing art of the common people rarely contains blanket statements such as, "In order to fight illness A, you must use treatments a, b, or c."

Some readers may look for a strict formula or prescription in this book, so they can follow a recipe exactly. I have to disappoint you there because blanket formulas simply do not exist in the science of folk healing.

Mechanistic thinking like this appeared much later. Old medicine views the human being as a whole, but also as a unique entity. As a result, it is clear that experience and the ability to be sensitive are of utmost importance in finding the right healing remedy. Both can be acquired—sometimes quickly, sometimes a little more slowly. Ultimately this is still true in the modern healing sciences, except that people tend to experiment more instead of using their intuition. If a patient does not respond to one type of medicine, he will receive another until something (hopefully) fits.

Magnetism is the healing power that rests within each person. In folk healing this term has nothing to do with either the physical phenomenon of magnetism or magnetic bracelets or any of those things. Today we'd call it energy or aura. Magnetism does not only describe healing power (exactly like our term for energy today), but also the basic energy of a person, meaning his or her strength, charisma and centeredness in their own power.

Magnetism further covers the topic of techniques that include laying on of hands and all other applications that allow healing energy to flow into the body of a patient. We call this energy "work" today. Only the terms have changed.

The terms used in folk traditions often display a shift in meaning. If we want to express it simply, sympathy and antipathy refer to healing through magic, plants, stones, and spells while magnetism requires an energy flow from the healer to the patient. Both are often applied at the same time. Of course, even a strictly herbal healer will also speak to her patients, which automatically triggers an exchange of energies between two people.

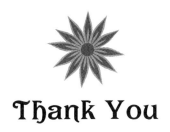

Thank You

I would like to thank all of those who share their knowledge and thus keep it alive. Keeping secrets benefits the individual; sharing knowledge benefits everyone.

I further send a heartfelt thank you to all of those people and spirits that have taught me to look ahead.

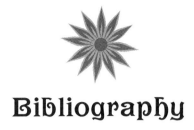

Bibliography

Arrowsmith, Nancy. *Field Guide to the Little People*. Llewellyn Publications, 2008.

Atkinson-Scarter, Dr. H. *Sympathiemagie und Zaubermedizin (Sympathetic Magic and Spell Medicine)*. Richard Schikowski Publishing, 1960.

Bauerreiß, Erwin. *Heimische Pflanzen der Götter (Our native Plants of the Gods)*. Raymond Martin Publishing, 1995.

Bitter, Wilhelm. *Magie und Wunder in der Heilkunde (Magic and Miracles in Medicine)*. Klett Publishing, 1959.

Brooke, Elisabeth. *A Woman's Book of Herbs*. Women's Press, 1999.

Bühring, Martina. *Heiler und Heilen (Healers and Healing)*. Reimer Publishing, 1993.

Derlon, Pierre. *Die geheime Heilkunst der Zigeuner (The Secret Art of Medicine of the Gypsies)*. Goldmann Publishing, 1978.

———. *Heiler und Hexer (Healers and Warlocks)*, Sphinx Publishing, 1984

Detterbeck, Pius. *ie Wirkung der Heilkräuter auf die wichtigsten Organe des Menschen (The effects of healing plants on major human organs)*. Kräuterhaus (Herbal House) Hamburg, publication date unknown.

Edenheiser, Iris. *Kallawaya Heilkunst in den Anden (Kallawaya—Healing Arts of the Andes)*. Grassi Museum for Ethnology Leipzig, 2010.

Favret-Saada, Jeanne. *Deadly Words: Witchcraft in the Bocage*. Cambridge University Press, 1981.

Fehrle, Eugen. *Zauber und Segen (Spells and Blessings)*. Eugen Diederichs Publishing, 1926.

Fillipetti, Herve and Janine Troterau. *Zauber, Riten und Symbole (Magic, Rites and Symbols)*. Hermann Bauer Publishing, 1992.

Frazer, James George. *The Golden Bough*. Dover Publications, 2002.

Frischbier, Hermann. *Hexenspruch und Zauberbann (Witch's Spell and Magic Charm)*. Enslin Publishing, 1870.

Gaßner, Franz. *Brauchtum und Aberglaube aus dem Brandenberg (Old Traditions and Superstitions from Brandenberg)*. Tiroler Heimatblätter (Tyrolese Homeland Pages), 1936..

Gessmann, G.W. *Die Pflanze im Zauberglauben (The Plant in magical Beliefs)*. J.J. Couvreur Publishing, publication date unknown.

Golowin, Sergius. *Das Reich des Schamanen (The Realm of Shamans)*. Goldmann Publishing, 1989.

Hampp, Irmgard. *Beschwörung Segen Gebet (Invocation, Blessing, Prayer)*. Silberburg Publishing, 1961.

Hanf, Walter. *Dörfliche Heiler, Gesundbeten und Laienmedizin in der Eifel (Rural Healers, Health Praying and Lay medicine in the Eifel region)*. Greven Publishing, 2009.

Höfler, Max. *Wald- und Baumkult in Beziehung zur Volksmedizin Oberbayerns (Forest and Tree Cult in Relation to Upper Bavarian Folk Medicine)*. Nabu Press, reprint from 1923.

Kindred, Glennie. *Herbal Healers*. Wooden Books, 1999.

Köstler, Gisela. *Wurzelsepp und Kräuterweibl (Root-seller and Herbal Woman)*. Kremayr & Scheriau Publishing, 1981.

———. *Geheimnis und Zauber im Alpenland (Secrets and Magic of the Alps)*. Styria Publishing, 1980.

Kronfeld, Dr. Moritz. *Zauberpflanzen und Amulette (Magic Plants and Amulets)*. Moritz Perles Publishing, 1898.

Leland, Charles Godfrey. *Gypsy Sorcery and Fortunetelling*. T. Fisher Unwin, 1891.

Liek, Erwin. *Das Wunder in der Heilkunde (The Miracle in Medical Science)*. Lehmanns Publishing, 1940.

Luppertz, Paul and Albert Spülbeck. *Lommersdorfer Chronik (Lommersdorfer Chronicle)*. Self-published, 1990.

Marinova, Marina. *Magie und Heilkraft der Kräuter (Magic and Healing Power of Herbs)*. Silberschnur Publishing, 2004.

Nemec, Helmut. *Zauberzeichen (Magic Signs)*. Schroll Publishing, 1976.

Nitz, Dido. *Kräuterzauber (Herbal Spell)*. arsEdition Publishing, 2012.

Paine, Sheila. *Amulets. Sacred Charms of Power and Protection*. Inner Traditions, 2004.

Parrinder, Geoffrey. *West African Religion*. Epworth Press, 1949.

Petzold, Leander. *Kleines Lexikon der Dämonen und Elementargeister (Little Dictionary of Demons and elemental Spirits)*. C.H. Beck Publishing, 1995.

Rudolph, Ebermut. *Die geheimnisvollen* Ärzte *(The mysterious Doctors)*. Walter Publishing, 1977.

Ruff, Margarethe. *Zauberpraktiken als Lebenshilfe (Magical Practices as Self-Help)*. Campus Publishing, 2003.

Scherf, Gertrud. *Zauberpflanzen Hexenkräuter (Magic Plants, Witch Herbs)*. BLV Publishing, 2003.

Schmelz, Bernd. *Hexerei, Magie und Volksmedizin (Sorcery, Magic and Folk Medicine)*. Holos Publishing, 1997.

Schmidt, Ingrid. *Orakel, Hexen, Heilmagie auf der Insel Rügen (Oracle, Witches, Healing Magic on the Island of Ruegen)*. Hinstorff Publishing, 2004.

Schöpf, Hans. *Zauberkräuter (Magic Herbs)*. Akademische Druck- u. Verlagsanstalt Publishing, 1986.

Seligmann, Dr. S.. *Die Zauberkraft des Auges und das Berufen (The magical Powers of the Eye and Ensorcellling)*. J. Couvreur Publishing, 1921.

The 6th and 7th Books of Moses (available from various publishers).

Speckmann, Hermann. *Besprechen im Oldenburger Land (Talking off illnesses in the Oldenburg region)*. Isensee Publishing, 2008.

Strackerjan, Ludwig. *Aberglaube und Sagen aus dem Herzogthum Oldenburg (Superstition and Legends from the Duchy of Oldenburg)*, Volume 1 and 2, Gerhard Stalling Publishing, 1867.

Tenhaeff, Wilhelm. *Aussergewöhnliche Heilkräfte (Exceptional Healing Powers)*. Walter Publishing, 1957.

Thenius, Erich. *Fossilien im Volksglauben und im Alltag (Fossils in folk Belief and daily Life)*. Waldemar Kramer Publishing, 1996.

Treben, Maria. *Health Through God's Pharmacy*. Ennsthaler Publishing, 2009.

Tscharner, Gisula and Heinz Knieriemen. *Hexentrank und Wiesenschmaus (Witch's Brew and Meadow Feast)*. AT Publishing, 2002.

Tschinag, Galsan. *Der singende Fels. Schamanismus, Heilkunde, Wissenschaft (The singing rock. Shamanism, Arts of Healing, Science)*. Unions Publishing, n.d.

Unger, Franz Xaver. *Die Pflanze als Zaubermittel (The Plant as Medium of Spells)*. Antiquariat Feucht Publishing, 1979, reprint from 1858.

Wagner, Johanna. *Ein Füllhorn göttlicher Kraft (A Cornucopia of divine Power)*. Clemens Zerling Publishing, 1992.

Wlislocki, Heinrich von. *Aus dem inneren Leben der Zigeuner (Insights from the Inner Life of the Gypsies)*. Emil Felber Publishing, 1892.

———. *Volksglaube und religiöser Brauch der Zigeuner (Folk Beliefs and Religious Customs of the Gypsies)*. Aschendorffsche Buchhandlung Publishing, 1891.

———. *Zauber- und Besprechungsformeln der transsilvanischen und südungarischen Zigeuner (Magic Formulas and Incantations of the Transylvanian and South-Hungarian Gypsies)*. The British Library, 2010.

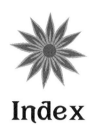

Index

protection, 22, 24, 28, 32, 78, 118, 135–137, 157, 183, 184, 186, 189, 190

psoriasis, 107, 135, 145

psychosomatic, 73, 186

quartz crystals, 26

rashes, 14, 21, 23, 97, 119, 120, 153, 154, 193

red stones, 31, 32, 136, 137, 188, 192, 195

strength, 22, 31, 35, 43, 47, 53, 55, 65, 69, 78, 79, 83, 85, 94, 103, 121, 124, 136, 137, 147, 155, 168, 169, 190, 206

relaxation, 145

rheumatism, 105, 114, 135, 148

right way, 47, 59

rock crystal, 26, 27

Rose, the, 23, 97, 120–122

rosemary, 108, 170, 171, 177

rose quartz, 26

rye, 43, 124

sage, 29, 162, 170, 171

salve, xi, 131, 142, 143, 145–147, 163, 177

Sara (la) Kali, 58, 59

Saturday, 67, 68

Saturn, 67, 72, 73, 159

scabby head, 155

scars, 95, 142

schnapps, 56, 111, 139, 140, 155

sea salt, 29, 107

second sight, 15, 16, 25, 51

sexual organs, 72

Sheela Na Gig, 45

shoulders, 5, 70, 117, 165

sickness spirits (see: worms)

To Write to the Author

If you wish to contact the author or would like more information about this book, please write to the author in care of Llewellyn Worldwide Ltd. and we will forward your request. Both the author and publisher appreciate hearing from you and learning of your enjoyment of this book and how it has helped you. Llewellyn Worldwide Ltd. cannot guarantee that every letter written to the author can be answered, but all will be forwarded. Please write to:

Hexe Claire
℅ Llewellyn Worldwide
2143 Wooddale Drive
Woodbury, MN 55125-2989

Please enclose a self-addressed stamped envelope for reply,
or $1.00 to cover costs. If outside the U.S.A., enclose
an international postal reply coupon.

Many of Llewellyn's authors have websites with additional information and resources. For more information, please visit our website at http://www.llewellyn.com